INTERMITTENT FASTING FOR WOMEN 101

THE COMPLETE GUIDE TO THE INTERMITTENT FASTING DIET FOR WOMEN. PROMOTE HEALTH AND WEIGHT LOSS THROUGH AUTOPHAGY. BONUS: FASTING FOR WOMEN OVER 50 AND KETO DIET.

By
ROSANNE MILLER

TABLE OF CONTENTS

INTRODUCTION 1
   The Science of The Human Body 1
CHAPTER 1. What Is Intermittent Fasting? 4
   So … What Is Intermittent Fasting? 4
   Intermittent Fasting For Human Survival 5
   Your Two Fasting Goals 7
   Are You Fasting Or Feeding? 8
   The 3 Types Of Intermittent Fasting 9
CHAPTER 2. Intermittent Fasting And Hormones 11
   Hormones & Health: Weight Loss 11
   IF & The Female Body 12
   Physical Effects Of IF For Women 13
   Using IF To Help With Periods, Fertility, And Metabolism 14
CHAPTER 3. Benefits Of Intermittent Fasting 16
   Weight Loss 16
   Reduces Insulin Resistance And Risk Of Type 2 Diabetes 17
   Cells, Genes, And Hormones 18
   Inflammation And Oxidative Stress 19
   Heart Health 19
   Cellular Repair 20
   Cancer 20
   Alzheimer's Disease 21
   Longevity 22
CHAPTER 4. Intermittent Fasting And Autophagy 23
   Does Autophagy Help Women? How? 30
   Does Autophagy Have Anti-Aging Effects Too? 30
   How Does Your Body Renew Itself Through Autophagy? 31
CHAPTER 5. Different Types Of Intermittent Fasting (16/8, 14/10, Etc…)
.... 33
   The 16/8 Method 33
   The Importance of Your Circadian Rhythm 35
   The 5:2 diet 35

Eat-Stop-Eat diet 36
Alternate day fasting 37
Warrior Diet 38
Spontaneous Meal Skipping 38
Extended Fasting 39
Why Should I Try Intermittent Fasting? 39
CHAPTER 6. What To Eat And What Not To Eat During Fasting 41
Food To Eat During Intermittent Fasting 41
Food Not To Eat During Intermittent Fasting 43
Side Effects Of Intermittent Fasting 44
CHAPTER 7. What To Drink And What Not To Drink During Fasting .. 47
CHAPTER 8. Differences Of Fasting Between Men And Women 53
Obesity And Its Impact On Women 53
The Crucial Role Of Cholesterol In A Woman's Life 54
Why Autophagy And Protein Cycling Matter Especially For Women ... 55
Hormonal Effect Of Fasting On Women 55
A Gentle Fasting Solution For Women 56
Symptoms You Should Watch For 57
During Menstruation 57
During Menopause 58
CHAPTER 9. Tips and Tricks For Intermittent Fasting 60
Incorporate Meal Prep 60
Figure Out Your Plan 61
Write Your Grocery List 62
Make Your Meals 62
Take Pictures And Measurements 63
Expect Ups And Downs 65
CHAPTER 10. Who Can Do Intermittent Fasting And Who Cannot 66
Who Should Fast? 66
Who Shouldn't Fast? 67
A Woman On Menstruation 68
A Woman On Menopause 72
CHAPTER 11. Intermittent Fasting For Pregnant Women 74
CHAPTER 12. A Proper Shopping List 79
Juices And Smoothies Recipes 83

- Centrifuge Detox 83
- Green Extract..or Meal! 83
- Red Juice 84
- Juice of the day! 84
- Strawberry Smoothie, Raspberries and Yogurt 85
- Recipe For Your Health 85
  - Magical Smoothie 86
  - Cheese Waffles 86
  - Salmon and Asparagus 87
  - Mushroom Pie 87
  - Pumpkin pie 88

CHAPTER 13. Diet For Intermittent Fasting 90
- Breakfast 90
- Lunch 92
- Dinner 93
- Snack Time 95
- Meal Plan 95

CHAPTER 14. Fasting For Women Over 50 97

CHAPTER 15. How To Implement With Keto Diet 104
- All About Ketosis 104
- Ketones Used As Fuel 105
- The Keto Macros 106
- Keto Approved Foods 107
- The Keto Diet And Intermittent Fasting 112

CHAPTER 16. 16 The Science Of Intermittent Fasting 113

CHAPTER 17. Everything You Need To Know About The Eat Stop Eat Program 121
- Can You Fast For 24 Hours? 121
- Is Cutting Down On Carbs Your New Meal Philosophy? 122
- How To Exercise During The Eat Stop Eat Program? 124

CONCLUSION 128

INTRODUCTION

Intermittent fasting refers to different eating plans that revolve within the cycle amid starvation as well as non-fasting for a given time. There exist three forms of intermittent starvation; Substitute Day Starvation, Time-controlled Feeding, and Complete Day Fasting.

When it comes down to it, females' abilities to carry their children within their bodies means that the body can very easily tell when the individual is starving, and it won't allow that person to have children at that time.

In the following pages, we will begin by describing the sciences of sex difference and nutrition, and then we will explore how these two things interact through a discussion about male vs. female bodies' reactions to hunger.

You should understand how IF will affect you because you're female, and you will likely still have a lot of questions about the procedure ahead of you. That curiosity is totally valid, and all your questions will be answered in time. To start, let's look at the science of the human body.

The Science of The Human Body

Have you ever wondered why it happens to be that you eat more when you're hungry than you're hungry for? Have you ever been curious about why you sometimes can't stop even when you know you're full? As someone coming to IF with goals of weight loss, you likely are very familiar with these frustrating feelings, but if you're coming to IF with goals other than weight loss, you might not be as familiar.

Regardless of your experience with hunger and whether or not you're able to stop eating when you feel you're full, there are scientific reasons why the saying "Your eyes were bigger than your stomach!" exists. First on this list of reasons is the existence of hormones leptin and ghrelin. Both leptin and ghrelin seem to have a large effect on regulating appetite, and subsequently controlling fat storage and gain.

While leptin is secreted from fat cells in the stomach, heart, skeletal muscle, and placenta in females, ghrelin is secreted basically only from the lining of the stomach. Despite where the hormones come from, however, they both end up affecting the brain. Leptin decreases feelings of hunger, while ghrelin does the opposite. Leptin and ghrelin both end up communicating with the hypothalamus in the brain about stopping or starting to eat, but their effects are divergent.

Insulin is another hormone that our bodies produce that effects our health in several ways. For instance, insulin is produced in the pancreas, and it helps regulate the amount of glucose in our blood, but if someone's insulin levels are too high or too low, his or her weight is imminently affected. With low insulin levels, one can't help but lose weight, but too low of insulin levels can be dangerous because the body needs sugar to use as energy. The trick is finding a healthy balance while working to lose weight.

If you're overweight or working with IF, your hormones' signals to the brain become affected. If you're obese, for instance, the signals are interrupted and distorted, while for those working with IF, those signals are triggered not to go off as frequently through an altered pattern of eating.

The thyroid regulates hormones that affect the speed of your metabolism, and if your thyroid is over- or under-worked, your health, energy level, and weight will certainly be affected. In order to lose weight, you'll want to speed up your metabolism without hurting or overworking your thyroid, and that can be tricky to work out properly sometimes.

How the Male vs. Female Bodies React to Hunger

When it comes to the science of the human body, everything matters, from the foods we eat to how often we eat, what hormones we allow to produce, which ones we limit, and how well our thyroids are working.

When you're hungry, your body sends signals to the vagus nerve in your brain, and it communicates a lot of details. It reveals how empty (or full) your stomach happens to be, the nutrients that are processed in the intestines, and what deficiencies may be present in the body as a whole. After the stomach sits empty, it starts to grumble (a process called "borborygmus," which pushes any remaining food into the intestines to be digested fully), and then your stomach and intestinal walls begin producing that hormone, ghrelin, that makes you feel hungry.

If you're female and you tell yourself you're not hungry when you get this feeling, your brain often doesn't work in your favor

CHAPTER 1.
What Is Intermittent Fasting?

Cool, so you want to add Intermittent Fasting to your life and not just shed those pesky pounds, but gain many other rewards along the way!

You definitely can.

We'll also examine some of the silly myths around fasting. I want to get you excited to start upon this journey!

So ... What Is Intermittent Fasting?

It is exactly what it sounds like!

When you do something intermittently, that means you are not doing it continuously, but in smaller amounts. To fast is to abstain from all foods that have calories for a certain period of time.

When you add those two words together, you get Intermittent Fasting!

This is a scheduled way of combining both extended fasting times and eating times into a continuous routine. It is a way to unlock the exciting features and benefits of Intermittent Fasting, which gives you incredible rewards like:

~A slimmer, trimmer body
~Amazing energy
~Better health
~Having your cells cleaned and revitalized

~Effortless weight loss

~No exercise required!

That is what Intermittent Fasting is designed to do.

But, why has this become a new way of losing weight? What makes it so powerful, and why is it an ideal process for your body to drop the pounds?

Those answers come from how your body actually works and has worked for centuries!

Intermittent Fasting For Human Survival

While in modern times, there is a grocery store or restaurant on every corner … that was definitely not the case throughout most of human history.

Picture this:

It is thirty thousand years ago, in Europe. It's at the height of summer, but winter is only a few months away. You are expending a lot of calories just doing your daily living. But you're also eating as much as you can while the plants are in season and the animals are plentiful. You eat and eat, basically gorging yourself and eating way more calories than you normally need to survive.

But thousands of years ago, that's exactly what was happening. Your body stored every tiny extra bit of nutrients in your fat cells. That was their purpose then, and it is still their purpose! You were meant to store extra fuel.

After a few months, the plants died, the animals became scarce, and winter came. Now your body was prepared to face the months and months of vastly reduced food supply. You had spent your summer days storing the food that you needed.

Winter was historically a months' long fasting period. Your body was prepared for it, and your ancestors survived those long, cold winters. You're here!

But your body was built to withstand prolonged fasting times with few calories to sustain you. You were forced to live off of the stored fuel. Consequently, your body switched metabolic states and went into what's called ketosis. Ketosis helped your body use fat as a primary fuel source, not glucose.

Our ancestors survived because their bodies could switch metabolic states so easily, adapt to pretty hardcore fasting, use their stored fuel efficiently, and prevent themselves from starving to death.

Nowadays, though, we live in seriously the most abundant and food plentiful time in human history. Our ancestors would be staggered at the amount of food available to us, the variety, and the constant freshness! They had to make do with whatever they could hunt or gather.

So, that is the history of fasting. It is built into the DNA of each of your cells. Your body was economically designed to conserve and store as much food as humanly possible. It is very efficient and has helped the human race persist and thrive as much as we have for thousands of years.

However, it certainly does not help modern humans like you and me who want to lose that conserved and stored energy! We want to shed that stored fuel, and we want to do it quickly.

The best way to do that?

Turn back the clock on your body. We are going to pretend like it is thirty thousand years ago. We want your body to go into a prolonged fasting mode, so that your existing stored fuel is used. The less stored fuel on your body, the less you weigh. Intermittent Fasting will help you meet those weight loss goals.

That's really all there is to it!

Your Two Fasting Goals

You have two basic goals with Intermittent Fasting:

~Burn even more fat than you would if you weren't fasting
~Boost your energy levels

When we proceed to the preparations before the 30 Day Challenge, you'll be thinking about the weight loss goals to set. It's great to set a small amount of weight to lose, but don't be surprised if your weight loss far surpasses that! Intermittent Fasting is specifically designed to burn fat. Many women have reported astonishing results. You will, too!

Imagine what you would be able to do if you did have plenty of extra energy. Right now, you're probably feeling sluggish from blood spike and crash cycles. Not to mention that your life is pretty busy. You have a full to-do list each day. How can you expect to get it all done?

That is when the power of Intermittent Fasting comes into play. This is an extremely energy boosting way of eating. It lifts up your energy levels to new heights, and helps you accomplish everything you need to do each day – and then some! Wouldn't it be great to feel younger, refreshed, vitalized, and having a natural positive outlook each day? Well, when you decide to both fast the correct way and eat the correct way on Intermittent Fasting schedules, that's really when great stuff happens.

Are You Fasting Or Feeding?

Intermittent Fasting is not just about abstaining from food. You are actually going to both eat and not eat on a continuous looping cycle. There are two parts to this cycle:

~Fasting times
~Feeding times (also known as eating windows)

You are either in one or the other.

You actually already implement a fasting cycle every day of your life! Did you know that? It's when you are sleeping in between dinner and breakfast. The word "breakfast" literally comes from the phrase "break a fast." Yes, sleeping definitely counts as fasting.

Most of us follow a pretty regular weekly feeding schedule of eating breakfast in the morning, lunch around noon, and dinner in the evening. You fast at night when you sleep. You feed and fast, feed and fast, continuously throughout the weeks and months.

With Intermittent Fasting, we are going to take that same schedule, but just apply more rigidity and structure to it. So, instead of being free to eat whenever you want while you're awake, now you'll have a set period of time when you are supposed to be eating. Also, instead of just fasting when you're asleep, you will also set aside certain hours during the day to fast while you are awake.

Creating your own feeding schedule means that you will set up what are called eating windows. You will be consuming all of that day's calories within the window of time.

Your Intermittent Fasting schedule is now entirely dependent on the clock! Are you feeding or fasting? Depending on the time of day and your Intermittent Fasting schedule, you will know.

The 3 Types Of Intermittent Fasting

There are three main types of Intermittent Fasting schedules. Let's take a look at them from easiest to the most challenging.

1. Skipping Meals

You have probably skipped breakfast many times before, especially if you were trying to get to class or work on time. You just did not know you were Intermittently Fasting at the same time. Skipping meals to extend a fast is definitely the easiest way to continue the benefits of fasting. You could either skip breakfast to extend your fast from the night before, or you could skip dinner to start your nightly fasting time earlier. When you skip meals, you reduce your eating window. You want to make sure you're hitting your calorie count goals before your next fast starts.

2. Fast a Lot, Eat a Little

This is the second most common type of Intermittent Fasting. You stick to a schedule that includes a long period of time fasting followed by a shorter eating window. These eating windows average between six and eight hours per day. Then, you spend the rest of the time fasting. The most common types of this fasting schedule include:

~8 hour eating window / 16 hour fasting
~7 hour eating window / 17 hour fasting
~6 hour eating window / 18 hour fasting

I'll talk a lot more about this version of Intermittent Fasting, because it is the most common and also helps produce amazing results!

3. Multi-Day Fasting

Once you get the hang of Intermittent Fasting and really want to take it to the next level, then you can try fasting for between 24 and up to 36 hours. This is a more complicated, complex version of fasting. You will need to prepare for it, and you will also need to have special mineral rich foods to eat once you come out of the fast, too. In the 30 Day Challenge, I have included two 24-hour long fasts. Those who do the multi-day fasting are especially pleased with the results.

CHAPTER 2.
Intermittent Fasting And Hormones

When you engage with IF as a woman, you will encounter struggles unique to your body. You may have to tweak your method, your timing, and your approach numerous times until you perfect your practice to what's the most healthy and productive for you.

You should feel more confident in how to alter your eating pattern to kick-start your metabolism without losing any of the good things your body does for you. You should feel interested in beginning or planning your lifelong intermittent fast.

Hormones & Health: Weight Loss

When it comes to female hormones, reproductive health takes internal and unspoken precedence over the weight concerns of the conscious individual. However, there have to be bigger biological reasons behind that increased sensitivity.

The cause seems to be kisspeptin, which is a molecule similar to a protein that helps neurons communicate with each other about hunger and energy and more. This molecule exists in both males and females, but females have far more kisspeptin than males do, making them even more sensitive to energetic changes in their internal balances.

Therefore, when females' bodies release hormones like leptin, ghrelin, and insulin (that make them feel hungry or full), their brains and internal systems are already that much more inclined to "hear" those feelings and respond to reestablish balance. Women are therefore more likely to struggle with weight loss and general health problems related to increased sensitivity. Despite your body's natural processes, however, you can absolutely learn how to make intermittent fasting work for you and still maintain your ideal weight, health, and productivity.

IF & The Female Body

Since intermittent fasting is not so much a diet as it is an altered pattern in eating times and frequency, its relationship with the female body is not the same as the standard diet's relationship would be. In fact, it's not necessarily supportive for females to practice a strict diet while intermittent fasting, for the combination of the two, can work serious havoc on the female body itself.

To counteract any curious side-effects of IF on your physical and mental states, you can try and make sure to eat as nutritious a selection of food as you can, whenever possible. Furthermore, you can try not to overexert yourself through exercise, especially since you're altering your food and nutrition intake significantly. Also, you can ensure that you're not forcing yourself to engage in IF if you're ill, suffering from an infection, or struggling with a chronic disorder of some kind. Finally, if your body is already exhausted from work or struggles with anxiety (or otherwise), you might not want to put yourself through additional stress with a new pattern of eating.

The most important thing to do as you begin to engage with intermittent fasting as a female-bodied person is to make sure you're as connected to (and introspective of) your body as you can be, as often as you're able to be. The more you know your body and its tendencies (i.e. the frequency of your period, your tendencies with metabolism, your fat storage areas, your most common moods, your emotional crutches, etc.), the more successful your experiences with intermittent fasting can be.

Physical Effects Of IF For Women

While the general effects of intermittent fasting include increased energy overall, clearer cognition and memory, improved immunity, slowed aging process, better heart health, increased insulin sensitivity, and more, are some of the physical effects for women deserve a little more detail in specific. For women, those specific details include:

lowered blood pressure in about two months or less, lowered cholesterol by ¼ the original toxic amount, better blood sugar control, decreased likelihood for type 2 diabetes, lowered chances of cancer, potential for increased muscle mass (with the ability to preserve it longer!), increased lifespan by up to 50 years, and increased awareness of internal bodily processes in general.

After a few months of intermittent fasting practice, you're sure to feel that your senses are somewhat heightened compared to how they were before, that your body works better and smoother than ever, that your weight melts off like wax from a candle, and that your mind and cognition are clearer than ever before.

Some physical effects function almost like warning signs for the woman practicing IF, too. If you experience poorer skin conditions, complete insomnia, loss of hair, excessive or shocking decrease in muscle mass, loss of period entirely, heart arrhythmia, or increased inflammations (whether internally or externally), you'll definitely want to consider altering your process, stopping the IF for a while, or visiting a nearby doctor for advice.

Using IF To Help With Periods, Fertility, And Metabolism

If you struggle monthly through painful periods; if you know you don't want to have children and you're not concerned about future fertility; or if you want to kick-start your metabolism to help yourself lose weight, all you have to do is start intermittently fasting without any concern whatsoever. If you're looking for hard and fast changes for your harsh menses, your fertility, or your weight issues, work your way up to fasting a few days a week, and you're sure to see the side-effects you seek played out within a month or two.

If you're interested in getting help with painful periods without substantial effects on your future fertility, simply make sure to get enough fat in your diet and supplemental estrogen (which you can find over the counter in a variety of forms). By making sure to consume enough healthy fat and by not restricting your caloric intake too much, you can use intermittent fasting to ease difficult menses without it having too much effect on your metabolism at the moment, and with it having hardly any effect on your fertility later on.

If you want the metabolism boost without effect on your periods or fertility, here's what you can do. Make sure you're eating enough healthy fats, but restrict caloric intake slightly, not too much though, mind you! You don't want to hurt those hunger hormones or inhibit your ability to ovulate and have a healthy period!

For these reasons, you should make sure not to intentionally or fastidiously "diet" while you're intermittently fasting but seeing as how you do want to lose weight and kick-start that metabolism, you can do something to help your body remember not to hang onto too much excess! That "something" that works so well is two-part: (1) once you define your method, keep to its timing strictly and; (2) when you have your meals, don't overindulge, binge, or gorge yourself; allow your caloric intake to be limited, but only slightly, as you work with IF.

CHAPTER 3.
Benefits Of Intermittent Fasting

In recent years there much by way of scientific evaluations has been done in intermittent fasting. This has demonstrated that intermittent fasting has a broad range of impressive health benefits. Not only can it help you to lose weight by using fat as energy, but it can also help prevent disease.

Weight Loss

The vast majority of people who try intermittent fasting are using it to help them lose weight. This works in two ways, firstly by reducing the number of overall calories being consumed, and secondly by improving hormone function that promotes weight loss.

This is due to the lowering of insulin levels along with the increase of norepinephrine, which is a growth hormone. This combination increases the metabolic rate and causes body fat to be broken down and used for energy.

The benefit of this double action is that weight loss is being promoted from two sides of the equation. The calories you are using are being increased, and the calories you are consuming are being reduced.

Most individuals see weight loss of between 3% and 8% over a three to twenty-four week period. If you look at it from another perspective and measure your waist circumference to gauge the amount of harmful belly fat lost, it can range between 4% and 7% in the same period.

Reduces Insulin Resistance And Risk Of Type 2 Diabetes

The instance of type 2 diabetes has shown a dramatic rise in recent years. This is thought to be mostly due to poor diet and the consumption of foods that cause insulin levels to become raised over long periods, causing firstly insulin resistance and eventually resulting in type 2 diabetes.

Our body's primary energy source is glucose, which we get from the food we eat. In recent times the amount of glucose-producing foods we consume has increased dramatically.

High carbohydrate processed foods are one of the biggest causes and include breakfast cereals, white bread, white pasta, white rice and products made with refined wheat flour such as cakes, cookies, and pastries. These foods are rapidly broken down into glucose in the body and the sheer volume that floods the system causes a big problem.

Having too much glucose in the bloodstream is bad news, and the body wants to use it up as fast as possible. To achieve this Insulin is released into the body, it helps it use up the glucose for energy and well as taking it to your liver, muscles and (if there is too much, which there usually is) your fat cells.

To give you the basic idea, insulin works by rushing around your body telling all the cells "Hey guys, look, there's lots of glucose here for you to use as energy!" At first, the cells respond and take in the glucose, but quickly they become full and don't want any more, so they start ignoring the message that the insulin is giving them. The body's reaction to this is to release more insulin to try to convince the cells to take the glucose. The insulin levels are raised higher and higher and over a period of time, you become insulin resistant. Eventually, this can lead to type 2 diabetes.

Intermittent fasting can reverse insulin resistance and reduce blood sugar levels, so avoiding type 2 diabetes and kidney damage.

Cells, Genes, And Hormones

Fasting causes your body to initiate a cellular repair process and changes hormone levels that allow body fat to be used as energy more easily.

This is what happens during fasting:

Insulin. The level of insulin in the blood drops significantly, allowing fat to be more easily used for energy.

Human Growth Hormone. The amount of human growth hormone circulating in the blood increases to up to 5 times the normal levels. This increase allows fat to be used as an energy source and muscle mass to be increased.

Cellular Repair. The cells of the body become more active, repairing themselves and eliminating waste materials.

Gene Expression. Due to the beneficial effects fasting has on gene expression and the function of hormones and cells, it is anticipated that intermittent fasting practices may not only protect against diseases but actually increase longevity.

Inflammation And Oxidative Stress

Many chronic diseases, as well as aging, can be promoted by oxidative stress. This is when free radicals, which are unstable molecules, interact with other important molecules such as proteins and even DNA, damaging them.

When combined with a diet that is high in antioxidant-rich foods, intermittent fasting may help your body be more resistant to oxidative stress.

Inflammation, which is a fundamental cause of many common diseases, can also be reduced by intermittent fasting.

A study published in the online issue 16 of Nature Medicine, describes how β-hydroxybutyrate inhibits a complex set of proteins known as inflammasome, particularly NLRP3. The inflammasome is responsible for driving inflammatory response in disorders such as type 2 diabetes, Alzheimer's disease, autoimmune diseases, atherosclerosis, and other autoinflammatory disorders.

Heart Health

The biggest killer in the world is currently heart disease. Intermittent fasting can improve many of the risk factors associated with heart disease, including LDL cholesterol levels, blood pressure, triglycerides, inflammation, and blood sugar levels. Making a useful way to help prevent the disease long term. This is particularly useful for people who have a family history of heart disease.

Unfortunately, because intermittent fasting is of no interest to the pharmaceutical industry (because they can't make money from it), very little study has been done on humans to ascertain the full effects that intermittent fasting can provide. To really understand the full potential a lot more human trials need to be done.

Cellular Repair

Cellular repair, known as autophagy, is stimulated by fasting. Autophagy is when all the dysfunctional and broken proteins that have accumulated within the cells over time are broken down and eliminated.

Autophagy can help protect the body against diseases such as Alzheimer's and cancer.

Cancer

Another disease that seems to have become more prevalent in recent times is cancer.

Cancer is the uncontrolled growth of cells, as the cells auto-destruct mechanism stops functioning and they continue to grow unhindered.

It is thought that when the body is in a fasting state that cancer cells cannot simply "wait out" the fast in the same way as normal cells do. Because they are permanently stuck in "on" mode, they cannot find the nutrients they need to sustain them during a fast. The healthy cells are unaffected, as they simply hibernate during the fast, which cancer cells cannot do.

Fasting is also useful for cancer prevention, as it reduces insulin resistance that is linked to several cancers. It also causes autophagy, where the cells clean out all the garbage, making them healthier.

As with heart disease, insufficient studies have been conducted to show the full potential of intermittent fasting in humans. We are now reliant on individual health associations to initiate the types of studies that are required to further prove the evidence gained to date.

The metabolic boost that intermittent fasting provides isn't only good for the body, it is good for the brain as well.

Oxidative stress, inflammation, blood sugar levels and insulin resistance all have negative effects on brain health. Intermittent fasting has been shown to generate new nerve cells that benefit brain function.

A brain hormone, brain-derived neurotrophic factor (BDNF) is increased with intermittent fasting. Deficiency in this hormone has been linked to depression and other mental health problems.

As intermittent fasting can also help to lower blood pressure to normal levels, it is helpful in the prevention of strokes and heart attack.

Alzheimer's Disease

Alzheimer's is the most common neurodegenerative disease and it is incurable. Prevention is, therefore, most definitely the best approach.

Patient's with Alzheimer's can benefit and show significant improvements when following short daily fasts.

Because fasting stimulates cell cleansing it is believed that it can help to prevent the occurrence of disease and maintain brain health.

Other neurological diseases such as Parkinson's and Huntington's may also be prevented or improved with intermittent fasting.

As with most other diseases, more scientific research on humans is required to show the full potential intermittent fasting could have

Longevity

Most of us want to live a long and healthy life, and intermittent fasting could be one of the keys to helping you achieve this.

Fasting has been shown to extend the lifespan of rats in the same way as continuous calorie restriction increases lifespan. It was shown in one study published in the Journal of Nutrition, Volume 31, Issue 3, 1 March 1946, Pages 363–375, that rats fasted every other day lived 83% longer than rats that did not fast.

Although more research is necessary on human subjects, intermittent fasting has shown to be greatly popular amongst the anti-aging crowd.

Due to the positive effects on health, it isn't difficult to understand how intermittent fasting can help with an increased lifespan.

CHAPTER 4.
Intermittent Fasting And Autophagy

Autophagy is the natural way your body disposes of toxic chemicals in your cells. You can't see it happening without a microscope, but your cells have been going through autophagy for your entire life without you ever noticing. In just the last twenty years, scientists have learned much about the metabolic process of autophagy. Most importantly for our purposes, they have learned more and more about how autophagy's implications for fighting against disease and aging.

The entire foundation of using intermittent fasting for losing weight and getting healthier is our current scientific understanding of autophagy. We know for a fact that autophagy can help us attain better general health and live longer. Autophagy isn't just for losing weight, however — although it does that job better than any other method. It used to be that people went through autophagy quite often. We went through autophagy more back in the days before industrial agriculture because we did not expect to have food all the time.

Nowadays in the industrialized world, most people rarely miss a meal. We always have food around us. But people back in the day did not even have an expectation to eat every single day. Our bodies went through advanced autophagy very regularly because of this. We can even say that our bodies are more built for not eating every day than they are for eating constantly as we do right now.

Our first encounter with autophagy in the world of science was thanks to the French scientist named Christian De Duve. He and a group of biologists took note of a bizarre organelle that they had never seen before; they named it the lysosome.

Before we knew all that we know now about autophagy, scientists thought that the lysosome was simply an organelle made for disposing of garbage. If you think about it, this doesn't even make logical sense, because there is not really such thing as disposing of something. You can change the form of something, but not dispose of it. If the lysosome were really an organelle that just kept breaking things down without recycling those parts, then eventually those tiny waste particles would build-up with nowhere to go.

Now we have an explanation for this problem because of autophagy, and this explanation has important takeaways for doctors, biologists, and anyone who cares about their health.

The Japanese scientist Yoshinori Ohsumi was the first scientist to get deeply interested in the lysosome of yeast cells. 2016 was the year he won the Nobel Prize when he learned that the lysosome was the center of a cellular process called autophagy. His key finding was that our cells never "dispose of" anything — they simply break down cellular waste into raw materials, and then use these materials to build new structures.

Ohsumi has created a new definition of autophagy. He says that autophagy is the way our cells break down waste materials for the purpose of freeing up space, killing harmful foreign toxins, and creating raw materials that can be used for building new cells. When Ohsumi first started, he was the first scientist to really have any interest in this topic. He started a scientific movement around autophagy when his research uncovered all the implications that autophagy has for our bodies. Not only did Ohsumi uncover much of our modern understanding of autophagy, but he was the one who coined the phrase "cell recycling." Cell recycling is what happens once autophagy is finished.

When your cells have cleaned themselves out, they use these raw materials for constructing things that other cells can use. They can also use these raw materials to create new cells if there is enough.

Now we know that autophagy can be considered the most important process for your cells both individually and collectively. Autophagy matters to your cells individually because it keeps them alive as well as possible; it matters collectively because your cells have to work together to be useful to your body as a whole, and autophagy keeps them working together smoothly when the process keeps them repaired and "cleaned out."

You also need to keep in mind the times that you should be eating these foods. The whole purpose of autophagy is lost if you eat during the times you are supposed to fast. That's because consuming anything puts your digestive system at work. When your body digests food, your autophagy stops. You need to really make sure you are not eating at all during these times that you have designated to be your fasting windows.

Even eating 20 calories disrupts autophagy entirely. You may think that eating a banana or a small snack during your fasting window won't change anything, but that isn't true at all. You would be shocked at how much changes in your body when you put food into it. The fact that so much changes is the reason why autophagy is so potent in the first place — because it is recovering from all the times that you were putting food into your body.

But How Does Your Body Know When To Start The Process Of Autophagy?

A signal must be sent to the organs to start breaking down the cells to produce energy. This can be done in many ways. It is not just fasting that can start autophagy in your body. Here are some other ways of losing weight that you can opt for.

Exercise

The more stress you create in the muscles and cells of your body, the more strongly the cellular cleanup phase will be triggered. All the extensive forms of exercise, including jogging, sprinting, weight training and physical training, regulate autophagy by inducing stress in the body. When the body is highly worked up, it needs energy that it gains by burning up the cellular waste.

Cold Showers

Yes, cold showers can also invoke healthy autophagy inside you. Studies have shown that people who swim during the winter exhibit higher levels of cell repair and recycling. Therefore, taking cold showers regularly can help you lose weight and stay healthy.

Steam Bath

Subjecting yourself to high temperatures through saunas and steam baths generates heat stress inside you. This heat results in the destruction and recycling of cancerous as well as damaged cells.

A trip to a spa can be good for relaxing, rejuvenating, losing weight and staying preventing diseases. Besides, exposing yourself to strong heat also helps to cure depression by naturally releasing heat shock proteins.

Intermittent Fasting

There are indicators in your body that activate or cease certain processes. The hormonal levels are one of them. When you begin intermittent fasting, you deprive the cells of essential nutrients. This activates the hormone glucagon in the body. This hormone works in opposition to insulin. While insulin increases blood sugar levels, glucagon brings them down to maintain the balance. The two hormones are like the ends of a see-saw.

When you are fasting, insulin levels go down, and, as a result, glucagon levels go up. This rise triggers autophagy. Your body gets the message that it is time to break down the stored fats in the body cells increase the insulin levels again.

Antioxidants

Though antioxidants do not directly invoke the process of autophagy in your body, they have been known to indirectly work towards it. Foods rich in antioxidants support the process when you are fasting, which in turn ensures that you undergo a healthy and balanced autophagy process.

Is There Something That Can Stop Autophagy?

There are factors that can stop your autophagy process. The major one is the mTOR. It stops the autophagy in your body when there are enough nutrients in the cells. It is highly sensitive and eating as little as 50 calories can increase the level of mTOR.

If you consume fats, it might not raise your insulin levels, and it might keep the mTOR levels suppressed. But high amounts of ketones and fats would break your fast.

Here is a list of things that you can take to keep your insulin levels low and let your body continue the waste removal process of your cells.

Green Tea
Coconut Oil
MCT Oil
Ginger compounds
Galangal
Reishi mushroom extracts
Black coffee
Apple cider vinegar

All these items can help to boost autophagy in your body.

Is It Just For Weight Loss?

Absolutely not. When the cells renew themselves by burning up the waste inside them, they do more than decrease your weight. Clean and healthy cells decrease the risk of developing diseases. Many forms of cancer, neurodegenerative diseases like Alzheimer's and Parkinson's, and metabolic and autoimmune diseases can be prevented through autophagy.

It helps fight infectious diseases and regulates inflammation. It has also been associated with fighting depression and schizophrenia. Fasting-induced autophagy is very helpful in keeping you healthy and preventing medical conditions. It is always good to get rid of the waste around and inside you. A clean environment is healthy and keeps you from getting sick.

Here is a list of major benefits of autophagy, both inside and outside of a body cell.

Increases metabolism

Decreases oxidative stress

Increases genomic stability that prevents cancer

Eliminates waste from the body

Increases neuroendocrine homeostasis

Decreases inflammation

Increases lifespan

Eliminates aging cells

Improves muscle performance

Does Autophagy Help Women? How?

The ghrelin or the hunger hormone increases more quickly in women than in men. Women start feeling hungry again quickly after having a meal. Their bodies start craving food much faster and, therefore, are under more stress to look for energy sources. The cleansing of their body cells makes them less immune to catching diseases and helps them to develop a stronger immune system.

Does Autophagy Have Anti-Aging Effects Too?

Consider a real-life example. Assume that you have two cars, X and Y. You are somehow biased towards car X, and so you take much better care of it. You wash it every day, get it serviced every few months, and refuel the tank. But car Y does not see many bright days. It is just a backup option for you for the days X is out for servicing or repairs. You do not get its tank refueled, it stays covered in dirt and has been for just one servicing in years.

Now, which car do you think would last longer? Obviously, car X. When you pay attention to health and get the repairs done on time, faults and damages do not pile up. Your car X would stay as good as new even after years of driving, but car Y would start causing trouble very soon.

The same thing happens with the cells in your body. When the non-functional components and cellular waste keeps sitting inside the cell, it degrades your health and makes you look older. But when they keep recycling and renewing, it shows on your skin. Rejuvenated and youthful cells make your skin softer and healthier.

Autophagy is like a cellular garbage disposal system. Newer cells wash away the dead and unhealthy ones. This leads to increased elimination of aging cells. Autophagy slows down the aging mechanism of your body that makes you look younger and healthier for a long time.

How Does Your Body Renew Itself Through Autophagy?

Small things matter, and when it comes to aging, small things are the only ones that matter. Cells are what keep you healthy and sick. They store energy, carry oxygen and do everything for your body. And they are the ones that keep you from aging on the inside and outside.

Let us understand how this works. The cells in your body are continuously at work, so they experience a lot of wear and tear. The over-used cells eventually stop working, thus becoming useless. When this happens, the production of new and healthy cells is also discouraged by the useless ones.

These used up cells are known as senescent cells. A senescent cell is a living cell, but its functioning does not contribute to maintaining person's health. And while they do not contribute to anything, they do not let new cells to get formed in the body either. Over the years, the senescent cells keep accumulating in the body. They perform just baseline functions, stop the creation of new cells and promote inflammation. The worst part for women is that they speed up the aging of the nearby cells.

Autophagy clears away the damaged cells, thus making way for the youthful cells to appear. You stay young, healthy and energetic for a long period. Therefore, working towards burning up the waste in your body cells is a great thing for you to do.

Developing healthy habits in your life is a good way to live. No one likes an untidy home; while a shining home with new furniture is loved by all, including the ones who live there. Autophagy is a way to throw away all the old things from home and make space for refreshing new things.

CHAPTER 5.
Different Types Of Intermittent Fasting (16/8, 14/10, Etc...)

The 16/8 Method

This is one of the most common methods that you can use in intermittent fasting. During this method you have to fast for about 14 to 16 hours each day, and eat the rest of the hours. During this feeding time, you can still take in two to three meals with no problem. This is more likely to fit in with the lunch schedule that you're used to, but it still affects you so you don't eat all day.

This approach is simpler than you'd expect. After dinner it's as easy as not eating meals and then skipping breakfast or at least having a late snack. Okay, you're just fasting for 16 hours because you're finishing your last meal at 8 o'clock in the night, and then eating nothing until midday the next day. Just be careful of the late-night therapies. Eating them in the morning will require you to skip coffee.

Many people have issues with this because in the morning they feel hungry for food and they know they need to sleep. Only shift the meal to a bit later in the day. If you choose, for example, to eat breakfast at 10 a.m. You would still be within the 16-hour period instead of eight, and then stop eating at 6 a.m.

As a woman, this form of intermittent fasting is advisable. With these shorter fasts, women typically do well and it is best to go fasting for 14 to 15 hours as this is more helpful to you.

During the quick, you are allowed to drink beer, tea, coffee and other non-caloric liquids to help lessen hunger pains. In fact, you should try to stick to healthier foods during your feeding time. Eating a lot of unsanitary food during this time isn't a good idea. Many people like to have a low-carb diet when they are on a fast intermittent because it deals with fatigue and gives better outcomes.

The rationale behind the approach of 16/8 focuses on your hormonal rhythms and biological clock. According to Satchidananda Panda, a professor at the Salk Institute for Biological Studies and an expert in the field of biology and circadian rhythms, the body has not only one biological clock but several which make up the full circadian rhythm. There's one biological clock in your liver, one in your kidneys and one in your stomach, and according to Panda, each of these clocks were switched on and turned off at various times.

Shortly after you feed the digestive system kicks in gear. When food moves through your digestive tract, every organ involved in the digestive process turns on, eats the food, and then turns off. When all digestive organs are shut off, it will allow the digestive system time to rest. During this time, the digestive system does its own "cleanup"—similar to a concept of a self-cleaning oven. Any remaining food residues are cleaned out, and the body is ready to start over again.

And if you constantly put food in your mouth, it will never shut down your digestive system, so it will never have enough time to perform its self-cleaning, which will have a negative impact on both your metabolism and overall health. Through his study, Panda found that giving the body an eight to twelve-hour, no-food window is best for your health. He claims it will help you lose weight (or maintain a healthy weight) and help stave off diabetes, high cholesterol and obesity by introducing a daily fasting period.

The Importance of Your Circadian Rhythm

For fully understand Panda's work, it is helpful to know what your circadian rhythm is, and how it affects the body. Also referred to as a body clock or biological clock, the circadian rhythm is a twenty-four-hour cycle that regulates many of the body's physiological processes, including sleep and digestion. The body gets signals from your circadian rhythm about when to go to sleep, when to wake up and when to feed.

Your circadian rhythm is regulated centrally by a brain area called the hypothalamus but is primarily influenced by natural, environmental signals such as temperature and light. For example, when it's dark outside, your eyes send a signal to your hypothalamus that it's time for you to sleep; your hypothalamus sends a message to the pineal gland (in another area of your brain) that activates melatonin (a hormone that helps you sleep), and you get sleepy. When it is light-out the opposite happens. Your eyes send your hypothalamus a signal, sending a signal to your pineal gland to reduce the production of melatonin. A dip in melatonin will make you stand up and get ready for the day.

The 5:2 diet

The 5:2 diet is another viable option. This fast advises you to eat normally for five days during the week and to limit yourself for each of the other two days to no more than 600 calories. This is sometimes called the Easy Diet, too.

It's recommended that on these fasting days, people will eat around 500 calories. You'll normally eat every day of the week, for example, and on Monday and Thursdays you'll have only two small meals with at least 500 calories. You can choose any day of the week as your fasting days, as long as you don't have them back to back. Choose your two busy days of the week, and make them fasting days.

There aren't many reports out there about the 5:2 diet, but it will provide most of the benefits you're finding as it's intermittent fast. You can do it without the need to think all day about making meals.

Eat-Stop-Eat diet

The Eat-Stop-Eat diet helps you skip 24-hour meals once or twice a week. This method was first popularized by Brad Pilon and has been a popular way to do the sporadic quickly for some time. You can do this quickly while still having one meal a day. Some citizens will have dinner every day, and then eat nothing until the supper of the next day. It lets you never go a whole day without eating but still collapsing in the 24-hour abstinence process.

You do want to change that though. You can choose one of those options when going from breakfast to breakfast or lunch to lunch is best for you. During your fast, you are allowed to have coffee, water, and other non-caloric drinks to keep you hydrated but you are not permitted to have any food at all.

Note that you're just fasting for one or two days a week. If it's time to eat properly, you need to consume the same amount of food you would have if you weren't on a fast. This will help you lose weight without hurting your body.

The only problem with getting on with this kind of erratic fast is that working for 24 hours is hard for most people. Nonetheless, you can ease that in it. You can find that beginning with a shorter speed, like the 16-hour fast, can produce some good results, and then continue to run for longer periods of time. Without food it can be hard to go through a whole day and most people tend to go with one of the other fasting options to see the same effects.

Alternate day fasting

With this choice, -alternate day you'll go on a fast. You can take with you a few things, and it depends on what applies to your needs. Some of those fasts that would allow you to have around 500 calories on your fasting days. You will find that most sporadic laboratory studies used some version of the simple alternate day to help determine all health benefits. Every other day it can be daunting to most people to fast.

It's certainly something you'll need to build up to every other day. It can be a struggle to push yourself to eat on alternate days. You'll probably feel very hungry many days a week on this fasting schedule, and it's hard to stick to that over the long run.

Warrior Diet

This is another popular option to choose from for intermittent fasting. It requires that you walk the entire day, eat just enough to keep you happy and then feast at night within a four-hour feeding window. The Warrior diet is one of the first diets to include a form of intermittent fasting.

Food choices which mimic the Paleo diet are also included in the warrior diet. Not only are you going to fast during most day and night events, but you are going to eat a diet full of unprocessed foods that look like what you see in nature.

Spontaneous Meal Skipping

You should do this if you want to prep your body for intermittent fasting, or if you don't want to spend a lot of time worrying about when you can drink. With this easy, you don't need to worry about following one of the more organized, intermittent fasting programs. You'll probably miss any meals occasionally. If you are not thirsty, or if you are too exhausted for a meal, you can do this. It is a big myth that you have to eat food every few hours to stop hunger.

The liver is well adapted without food, to last long periods. Waiting on a few meals isn't harmful to your health, particularly if you're not hungry or too busy.

If you end up eating a meal, or two, you are actually fasting. If you are too busy to get a snack out of the door just make sure you eat a good lunch and dinner. When you run out of errands and can't find a place to eat, then it's great to miss out on a snack. It will do no good and will really save you money.

You probably won't see results as good as some of the other options, but it's better than nothing and it's much easier to work with. Perhaps try skipping one or two meals during the week, or missing any meals when it's going for you.

As you can see, there are several different options you can deal with when you're ready to go on the sporadic quick. Some of these will be simpler than others and some will fit your timetable better. You'll need to choose which pace to work in your everyday life is best.

Extended Fasting

Although extended fasting belongs to one class of its own, it is important to understand the difference between it and the other types of intermittent fasting. Extended fasting is any form of fast that lasts longer than 24 hours. Long fasting can often last for a week and many of these long fasts simply require drinking liquids.

These types of fasts are more normal throughout the medical and surgical settings and are usually done when the body needs to experience substantial recovery or when the ability to feed is impaired. Without the guidance and monitoring of a medical professional, you should not pursue a continuous pace.

Why Should I Try Intermittent Fasting?

1. Reduces insulin resistance: Fasting is one of the most effective ways to restore the insulin receptors to a normal level.

2. Autophagy: This is the wonderful way the cells can "eat themselves" to get rid of damaged cells and replace the younger elements. Autophagy is also the mechanism by which foreign invaders such as viruses, bacteria, and other organisms are killed. Another method is apoptosis on regeneration of the whole cell. Without this process, the cancer risk increases, as damaged cells continue replicating.
3. Detoxification: Most of us have had prolonged access to diet and climate pollutants. Most of those are contained in our bodies ' fat cells. Fasting is one of the most powerful ways the body can absorb toxins.
4. Circadian Rhythms: The internal clock of your body regulates almost every process in your body and a cascade of negative effects can occur when it is disrupted. You reset the circadian clock, if you take a break from feeding.
5. Gut health: Fasting gives you the opportunity to refresh your digestive system and gut flora. This is significant, because the health of your digestive system regulates your immune system. There's more and more evidence that our moods and mental health co-depend on our gut microbiome.
6. Weight loss: Not necessarily, weight loss is improved by fasting. It also decreases insulin levels so the body won't receive the warning to retain extra calories as fat any more.
7. Heart function: With their high energy demands the heart cells can use fats, sugars, ketones and amino acids. Ketones have a metabolic role in fine tuning that optimizes cardiac output and protects the heart from inflammation and injury.

CHAPTER 6.
What To Eat And What Not To Eat During Fasting

Food To Eat During Intermittent Fasting

There is no specific rule that restricts people from eating whatever they want during intermittent fasting. The focus here is when you eat, not what you eat. However, it is not advisable to eat any food available or that you have a craving for. For intermittent fasting to be beneficial to your body, you have to complement it with your diet. Get into the habit of eating well-balanced diets that are full of necessary and useful nutrients. A balanced diet is usually essential, especially if you want to lose weight and maintain your focus throughout the intermittent fasting process.

Foods that should be consumed during intermittent fasting include:

- Water. It helps keep the body hydrated. Water is essential for the whole body and its organs to function. Drinking water is not an option, though most people take it as one. Not taking enough of it causes dehydration, which in turn results in light-headedness, fatigue, and headaches. Dehydration during fasting can have serious negative implications on your health. People drink different amounts of water. If you want to know whether you drink enough water, observe your urine. Urine should be a pale-yellowcolor. If it is dark, then your body is dehydrated.

- Avocado. Avocado is the fruit with the highest number of calories. Encouraging people to eat avocados is ironic because we try to lose weight by eating fewer calories. However, the monounsaturated fats in this fruit are highly satisfactory. According to a recent study, avocados help you feel full for longer hours than if you did not take it. It helps keep the hunger pangs at bay.
- Fish. Nutritionists suggest taking a minimum of eight ounces every week. Fish is a good source of vitamin D, protein, and healthy fats. Also, fish is sometimes referred to as brain food. Fasting can, at times, cause brain fog or destabilize your cognition. Eating fish will help you get rid of these effects.
- Cruciferous vegetables. A good variety of vegetables are rich in fiber. Fiber helps in the regulation and prevention of constipation. It also allows you to feel full for longer hours. These vegetables include cauliflower, Brussel sprouts, lettuce, and broccoli.
- Potatoes. We are often told that white foods are bad for our health. They are either not nutritious enough or have a significant amount of carbs. Potatoes are, however, one of the few white foods that do not fit in this category. They are highly satisfactory and can keep you full for long periods. They are also helpful in losing weight. This list does not include all potato products, such as French fries.
- Beans and legumes. Foods that contain carbs usually supply energy to the body. Intermittent fasting is about reducing your intake of carbs and calories, but it does not hurt to have carbs with low calories in your diet. Moreover, some legumes are

known to help reduce the weight of the body without restricting calories. These legumes include lentils, peas, black beans, and chickpeas.

- Probiotics. Probiotics are helpful bacteria that are good for the digestive system. Foods rich in probiotics include kraut or kombucha. They are used by the body to dispel the side effects of an unhappy gut. Your gut is not usually pleased when it does not receive food regularly. It causes specific effects on your body, like constipation. Probiotics help reduce these effects.
- Berries. Most berries, especially strawberries, are rich in vitamin C, which helps boost the immunity system of the body. Berries also increase the BMI of a person over a given period.
- Eggs. Eggs are one of the easiest foods to cook. They are rich in protein and help maintain muscle mass during fasting. They are also fulfilling foods, in that, you feel full for more extended periods after eating them.
- Nuts. Even though nuts contain a high number of calories, they also contain good fat. They have polyunsaturated fat, which changes the physiology of hunger.
- Whole grains. These are foods rich in proteins and fiber. They help in keeping you full after you've eaten. They also increase your metabolism rate. Examples of whole grains are sorghum, millet, spelt, and farro.

Food Not To Eat During Intermittent Fasting

Though intermittent fasting is not about what you eat, it is advisable to avoid certain foods are you partake in this practice. Avoid:

- Sweetened juice
- Sugary soda
- Simple carbs
- Sweets
- Processed foods
- Fast foods

Side Effects Of Intermittent Fasting

There has not been sufficient long-term research on intermittent fasting for everyone to be 100% certain of its benefits. It is clear that it has beneficial effects on the human body, but there are also risks involved when practicing intermittent fasting.

Health risks

Everyone should consult their doctor before beginning intermittent fasting, especially if the person is highly perceptible to health issues. Health problems are an issue associated with fasting among aged people or those with an existing illness or condition. Since this book mainly targets women over 50 years of age, it is advisable to seek medical consultation before embarking on this journey.

People on medication should consult their doctors before fasting. Usually, medicines are taken within the timeframe of eating, and fasting affects this timeframe. Moreover, if your work involves heavy lifting or other strenuous tasks, you will be at risk of getting dizzy spells, feeling lightheaded, or even having low blood sugar.

Fasting is not recommended for people with high caloric needs; that is, being underweight, pregnant, or younger than 18. Those with diabetes should also avoid fasting altogether. Fasting reduces your levels of insulin and blood sugar, which is dangerous for people with diabetes.

Developing an eating disorder is a high risk that comes with fasting. If you are likely to develop such a disorder, you should not fast in the first place. Restrictions on a diet can lead to these disorders for people with various risk factors. These risk factors include mood instability, having a close relative or friend suffering from an eating disorder, impulsivity, and being a perfectionist.

Feeling hungry

Feeling hungry is a common side effect of fasting. It distracts you from your fasting program. If the hunger pangs are too intense, it might lead you to forget the fast altogether and resume your old eating habits.

Overeating

Many people tend to engage in binge eating during non-fast days. Fasting can increase stress hormones, which cause food cravings. Once you give in to these cravings, you begin to overeat during your eating window. This is especially harmful if you are trying to lose weight because overeating increases your calories, resulting in gaining weight.

Dehydration

When not eating, people forget to give other body cues attention, more so thirst. In an attempt to not think about eating, they also forget to drink water, which leads to dehydration.

Tiredness

It is common to experience fatigue while fasting, especially newbies. Since fasting increases stress hormones, and the body already has low energy, sleep patterns tend to be disrupted. Lack of enough sleep during fasting days will most likely drain a person.

Irritability

Fasting affects your appetite, which in turn affects your mood. It is advisable to have a nutritionally balanced diet while fasting and getting enough sleep. This will help improve your mood.

CHAPTER 7.
What To Drink And What Not To Drink During Fasting

Cleansing and detoxifying the skin is essential. The first thing I want to know when someone asks me about this matter is what they want to clean/disinfect precisely. Maybe they are trying to lose weight, due to alcohol, heavy metals, to get away from drugs, to get rid of the metabolic waste, and caffeine. The purpose you purify defines the form you will have to use and quite often cleansing isn't necessarily to achieve a health goal. Maybe you aim to get more energy, and the reason you do not have high energy levels is that you have a nutritional deficit or an endocrine imbalance. Before you choose a method, you need to know the reasons behind the symptoms.

Caloric limits have the benefits of optimal health and intermittent fasting, in particular, to slow down aging biological processes. But it's hard to implement such techniques in a world full of calorie-rich, low nutrient foods and a society that insists on food every hour of the day.

We do not have to eat small mini-meals all day long, unlike common myths, to stabilize blood sugar, speed metabolism, and a slender physique. This day-long snack practice destroys your levels of blood sugar and insulin and allows them to rise and fall all day, even if you snack on "healthy" mini foods that contain a small amount of protein, fat, and fiber. Ideally, you want your insulin and blood sugar to rise as much as possible for a FEW times a day. This means eating only 2 or 3 meals a day, no snacks.

It is essential to reduce the frequency of eating between meals, when you consume snacks, to only 2 to 3 times a day before you go into the practice of intermittent fasting. It could take some days for your body to adjust to eating two or three times a day, during which you will experience symptoms of jittery, weakness, headaches, or nausea. This happens because you have trained your body to ask for a constant energy supply of food with eating a few mini-meals during the day instead of using glycogen stores in your liver and muscles (and eventually fatty acid storage from your fat cells) for energy. You cannot use your glucometers for energy because the constant supply of calories gradually produces a lenient liver (and a sensation of weightlessness and heaviness), which is why it is vital to use glycogen energy regularly.

The most effective way to purify the liver is not to take special "liver cleansing" pills, to wash salts/olive oil, or to take laxatives or enemas. The best way of cleansing the liver by allowing it to deplete its glycogen storage is to use water for a short time quickly! Your liver will store between 250-500 calories in the form of glycogen depending on your body's size, to be used when all calories have been used up. Depending on your body size, your muscles will store 800-2000 calories as glycogen. These glycogen stores in your liver and muscles are used for energy before your body starts mobilizing stored fat for energy. Fasting on water for 24-48 hours once or every second week can increase energy levels, offer huge anti-aging benefits, improved sleep quality and enhance the performance of sports, safely rest your body from digestion and allow your liver and muscles to purify themselves and detoxify themselves.

Juice Fasting is another great way of relaxing, cleaning, and restoring the body through a healthy seasonal juice. Juice fasting rapidly enters the mainstream, as specific juice cleaning programs and raw food restaurants have made it easy for people who for their own reasons can't make a juice at home to make a fresh juice on a regular basis each day. One thing you should watch out for in the juice-based program is that they rely heavily upon high-glycemic fruit juices that are high in calories, fat, or fiber, including possible added sweeteners such as honey or agave when they are prepared at a shop. This has the opposite effect which is calorie depletion and a minimal impact on blood sugar. The diet of fruit juice can cause candida yeast to be overgrown in the digestive tract, causing systemic yeast and associated symptoms of health such as exhaustion, nausea, gaining weight, brain fog, skin problems, and persistent vaginal yeast infections.

If you're interested in preparing your seasonal juice, you can buy your juicer to save some money and prepare your own customized vegetable juice recipes. If you are not seriously ill, juice cleansing can be very safe and beneficial to your health for a period of 3 to 10 days. During this time, you should be able to do your usual daily activities, although additional rest and light exercise are recommended. Always listen to and respect what your body says, and, if you feel extreme pain in any fasting or cleansing program, don't continue fasting until you are under direct medical control from a medical specialist qualified in fasting supervision.

Metabolism Boost

- 1 tablespoon of broccoli sprouts

- 1 tablespoon of laciniate
- 1 1/2 tablespoon of roman salad
- 1/3 of tablespoon of celery leaves
- 1 tablespoon of tomato
- 1/4 of a cup of red and yellow bell pepper
- 1 slice of cayenne pepper
- 2 tablespoon coconut oil
- 1 tablespoon MSM Crystals
- 1 raw egg

Directions

Take broccoli sprouts, laciniate, roman salad, celery leaves, tomato, red and yellow bell pepper, cayenne pepper, MSM Crystals, raw egg, put all in a food processor or mixer and mix the juice with the coconut oil.

Yield

- Get yourself to drink and feel the burn!

Morning Energizer

- 1/2 cup of roman lettuce
- 1/2 cup of coconut oil
- 1/2 cucumber• one beet
- five celery leaf
- 1/2 cup of ginger slice
- 1 tsp cocoa
- 1 tsp of cocoon

- 5-8 drops of a candida cleanse
- 1/2 cup of ginger

Directions

Take roman lettuce, cucumber, celery leaf, ginger slice, cocoa, cocoon, candida cleanse, ginger, put all in a food processor or mixer and mix the juice with the coconut oil.

Yield

- Get yourself a drink and feel the burn!

High-quality probiotics such as life colloids, which contain zeolites and lithophilic earth minerals to reprogram mineral cells, will boost detoxification of all your body's mycotoxins.

Also, keep in mind that using a far-infrared sauna allows your body to release accumulated toxins from your body's tissues through your sweat. The water also increases your central body temperature, which boosts your basal metabolic rate to facilitate fat loss and a variety of diseases.

Fasting is an excellent way to detox, to lose weight, and improve their health. Unfortunately, it is often difficult for most people living in our fast-growing society to spend time changing their habits and learn how to do so quickly. It's also a slightly intimidating process. The 24-hour fasting is an easy way to solve these problems! This is a great way to try fasting. It's also perfect for your overall health. Let's talk about it in more detail.

Fasting is achieved in two primary ways: 1) Fasting with water, and 2) Fasting with concentration. Water fasting is only recommended for professional fasters. Fasting juice is much more user-friendly and very effective. People can fast anywhere from one to thirty days, but some people go even longer. For most people, a fast 1-3 day is the best way to go, which will significantly benefit you. Some even benefit from fasting partially a day, like a 12 hour fast overnight. The critical aspect of juice fasting is to not eat solid foods, only liquids. It gives your organism a rest from the digestion of solid food that takes a lot of energy. Fasting does three essential things.

1. It helps clean up your body's toxin system.
2. It may help relieve the effects of a disease
3. kick your body into good health.

The juice is packed with vitamins and nutrients, especially organic and vegetable juices that are non-pasteurized. Green juices while fasting are highly recommended. The citrus extract can also be perfect for fasting, in particular, lemon juice. Some use cranberry juice, another good cleanser. Juice contributes to the purification process and also provides you with energy and essential nutrients. The juice is easy to digest for the liver, making it ideal for fasting.

CHAPTER 8.
Differences Of Fasting Between Men And Women

Can women fast? The short answer is yes, absolutely. The long answer is that pregnant and nursing women should never fast and women who do fast should watch for uncomfortable symptoms. If you don't feel right, visit the doctor and cease fasting. Your body will let you know if something is wrong.

Women and men both respond to fasting well. However, women tend to respond to longer fasts better simply because they have more experience dieting. Women will lose less weight than men in the first two weeks, but they will catch up in the next four to six weeks. Many women do not always shed pounds on IF, either, but rather they notice more muscle mass and a better fit for their clothes. The number on the scale is not an indicator of successful weight loss.

Women who fast also often report positive hormonal changes. They have fewer ugly period symptoms, less brain fog, elevated moods, and better sex lives, certainly a win for women! The fact that autophagy can repel cancer by cleaning out damaged and mutated cells can also help women to stave off breast, ovarian, and cervical cancer worries.

Obesity And Its Impact On Women

Obesity is obviously not good for anyone. But for women, it can be especially disastrous because of its effect on female hormones. Fat cells produce their own estrogen. This estrogen can become excessive, preventing proper progesterone production and upsetting the HPG axis, a delicate balance between hormones and the pituitary gland and the ovaries that regulates a woman's hormones and reproductive ability, as well as her endocrinological systems and moods. The result is that women will develop a hormonal imbalance called estrogen dominance, leading to issues like endometriosis, cysts, trouble ovulating, weight gain, trouble sleeping, poor mood control, irregular or absent periods, heavy periods, and trouble sustaining pregnancy.

Obesity also creates insulin resistance, which leads to more insulin production and more insulin resistance. The excess insulin triggers ghrelin and leptin, the hormones that stimulate hunger. The result is increased weight gain and a drive to eat more, that causes more weight gain. It is a vicious cycle, out of which many women struggle. IF can help with these issues by increasing insulin sensitivity and controlling hunger, while also removing the fat that produces too much estrogen.

The Crucial Role Of Cholesterol In A Woman's Life

Studies suggest that women need cholesterol, a wax that coats the veins, even more than men do. Women use cholesterol to manufacture estrogen, progesterone, bile acids, and vitamin D. While the last two elements are essential for every human being, the first two hormones are key to a woman's reproductive health. She will not be able to release eggs, ovulate, possibly get pregnant, and then stop menstruation and hold onto the fertilized egg without healthy cholesterol.

But because women need cholesterol, their bodies tend to make more of it and hold onto it more vigorously. Most women have elevated cholesterol and high cholesterol after menopause. High cholesterol will clog arteries, leading to heart strain and eventual heart trouble. It can also lead to visceral fat, dangerous fat that coats the organs and prevents healthy organ functioning.

Why Autophagy And Protein Cycling Matter Especially For Women

For women, the processes of protein cycling and autophagy are particularly important. Why is that? Because women are at risk for more types of cancer, with which fasting can help. Women tend to hold onto fat, which is disruptive to their hormones.

Now let's talk about protein cycling. Your body cannot create its own protein, so it must obtain protein from food sources. Women especially need protein to help burn fat and support hormonal health. Protein also satiates women, helping them to overcome the cravings that tend to destroy their ability to sustain fasting. Thus, an ideal approach involves eating lots of protein during eating windows and then fasting for up to 24 hours. This approach results in significant fat loss of up to ten percent.

Hormonal Effect Of Fasting On Women

Women have more of a hormone called kisspeptin, which makes them much more sensitive to fasting than men. They may also have more cortisol, which negatively influences their sleep cycles. Both of these hormones can cause a disruption in the HPG Axis, which will adversely affect the production of estrogen and progesterone.

Therefore, women should start fasting lightly. Then they should try a gentler approach. They should also exercise only lightly on their periods and on fasting days. These approaches will help reduce the possible bad side effects of IF. Generally, once women get used to fasting, they find that it helps them to balance hormones, sleep better, and handle stress so much better because it actually balances their HPG Axis.

A Gentle Fasting Solution For Women

The best approach to fasting for women is to fast for 24 hours once or twice a week, or in other words, use 5:2 fasting. Then on eating days, women should load up on healthy sources of protein from plants and animals and nuts.

Women should also ease into fasting. Start with a 12-hour fast, move to 16:8, then try 5:2. Be sure to have bone broth on hand for protein and craving satiation during fasting. Only exercise when you feel well enough to do so. Do not push your body. Lightly exercise on fasting days or on your period. On period days, you must consume at least 500 calories and be sure to eat lots of iron-rich foods.

Eating enough calories is very important. If the body goes into starvation, it will turn off reproduction first, and hormones can be disrupted for a long time or even permanently. This situation is why anorexic women typically lose the ability to get pregnant. Thus, you absolutely must eat sufficient calories in your eating windows.

Symptoms You Should Watch For

Any symptom that is so troubling it interferes with your quality of life is an issue for women. You should stop fasting and see a doctor if you experience any of the following symptoms:

- Unusual pelvic pain
- Bleeding with sex
- Unusual tiredness
- Pale skin
- Hair loss
- Weight gain
- Extreme weight loss (more than two pounds a week)
- Rashes on the skin
- Amenorrhea (the absence of a period for three months)
- Unusually painful and/or heavy periods
- Migraines
- Dizziness
- Fainting
- Vomiting
- Severe stomach pain

During Menstruation

Fasting will disrupt a woman's cycle, plain and simple. For menstruating women, this can mean that you stop your period. This disruption is only temporary until the body starts getting the nutrition it needs again. It is a reflex reaction to stress, which is the natural byproduct of fasting. IF will eventually lead to greater hormonal balance in women, if proper diet is practiced during eating windows. There is usually an adjustment phase that can be more noticeable in women who have more obvious signs of hormones such as menstruation.

Some women who engage in IF will discover pale skin, hair loss, missed periods, early onset menopause, and other hormonal issues. These issues usually subside in a few months if IF is appropriately practiced. That means not starving yourself for days on end, listening to your body, and eating a well-balanced diet with sufficient calories when in your eating windows. It also calls for taking a good multivitamin and listening to your doctor.

Menstruation is simply the expulsion of blood when your body does not detect pregnancy. Fasting does not necessarily affect it. Anecdotally, many women report fewer cramps and lighter bleeding during their periods, if they fast. It is your choice if you want to fast during your period or not. Often, women feel hungrier during their periods so you can forego fasting if it feels most comfortable for you. If you do decide to fast, be sure to eat more iron-rich foods, such as spinach and beef, and focus on more protein when you are in your eating windows.

During Menopause

Few studies show whether or not menopausal women should actually fast. Dr. Becky Gillapsy conducted a meta-review of studies done on fasting, women's health, and even getting older. The results she found are that women experience fasting no differently than men, even menopausal women.

Menopause often signals for the body to stop producing certain hormones, which can accelerate health problems and aging. Fasting can help the body mitigate these issues through autophagy. Higher risks of breast cancer are a problem that menopausal women face, which can be eliminated by IF. Alzheimer's can also be avoided.

CHAPTER 9.
Tips and Tricks For Intermittent Fasting

The most important thing that you can do is to have a plan to ensure your success with intermittent fasting. The first step is to decide what sort of fasting you'll do. Once that method of fasting has been decided, make a timetable. Can you fast every day? Which times are you going to fly, and what times are you going to be feeding? After you've established a schedule, another critical component will decide what you'll eat when it's time to get into your fed. Should you follow a specific dietary routine (such as the ketogenic diet or Paleo diet) or will you adhere to a simple clean-eating schedule without any particular "rules"?

Incorporate Meal Prep

Getting the basics down, planning your meals will help keep you on track and prevent you from getting into temptation for an unhealthy meal. Research shows that people who prepare their meals in advance experience greater success in their health and nutrition plans as well as long-term gains in time and money. You will make adjustments to your menus and your prepping schedule as you follow the rhythm of intermittent fasting and a new way of life.

Meal-Prepping Tips

One of the most important components of good meal preparation is getting organized. It may seem difficult to sit down and arrange meals and type everything out, or like a waste of time, but it will eventually save you hours down the road.

The amount of food that you make in advance and the amount of time you spend preparing is solely your responsibility. Many people spend three to four hours prepping meals on Sunday for the whole week. Many spend a few hours on Sunday preparing meals for the next few days, and then spend a couple more hours on Wednesday preparing meals for the remainder of the week. Whatever type of meal you select, organizing is important.

Figure Out Your Plan

You'll need to build your meal plan first. You should schedule a couple of days, a week or even the whole month. Find simple recipes, then write down what you're going to eat and when. The excitement may tempt you to look for fancy, new recipes or a lot of variety when you start with intermittent fasting and meal planning, but when you're in the initial stages of a new lifestyle change, one of the most beneficial things you can do is stick to the basics and not overcomplicate things.

Stick to foods you're already familiar with and recipes that won't take too long to prepare or require you to learn new cooking skills or purchase new cooking tools. After you get used to the basics and adjust your body and mind to the changes, there is plenty of time for you to try new things. The point of prepping your meal is to make you feel less stressed, and not add unnecessary tension.

There are online menu plans and trackers, as well as phone apps that you can use to keep track of your meals, but if automation is not your thing, you don't need any advanced gadgets or devices. Recording everything in a journal will keep it simple.

Write Your Grocery List

Once you've got your recipes together and written out your meal plan, it's time to figure out what you need. Before you write your grocery list, check your refrigerator and pantry so you don't buy things you already have. After compiling a list of things you've got on hand, write a list of the remaining items you'll need to complete your weekly recipes and meals (or for whatever length of time you've selected).

Through arranging your list of groceries based on where products are sold in the store you can save even more time. You can list all the meats together; together you can manufacture all the items and all the refrigerated items. For any deals or specialty items, organize your lists by store, if you need to go to different stores.

Make Your Meals

A great way to save money is to go shopping the same day you'll be preparing your meals. This way, when you get home, you won't have to put away as many food items— you can jump right into preparing your meals. Divide them into separate containers by portion size until the meals are prepared, and name them accordingly. So when you're ready to eat you're going to have a lunch ready to go and if you're bringing a food with you on the go it's going to be easy to bring.

Take Pictures And Measurements

If weight loss is one of your targets, don't rely on the scale alone. Your actual weight will fluctuate significantly from day to day, and even when your body is going through a huge transition, you might not see big changes in the figures. You can use the scale as a tool, but use a grain of salt to take those daily numbers.

Rather, take the pictures "before" and "after" (or "progress"). You should compare them side by side down the line, to see how the body has changed over time. Photos can be a really motivational device because you may not note the small changes happening when you see yourself every day but when you compare pictures taken a month ago, the changes may be much more noticeable. Don't allow any current body dissatisfaction to stop you from taking pictures beforehand. You are going to be happy that you have them down the road.

In addition to the images, taking body measurements is useful. You can start building leaner muscle mass, particularly if you regularly work out or carry out strength training. You may not feel too much of a difference on the scale when your weight starts to change but your body composition may change dramatically. Measurements can help you track progress by tracking lost inches from various areas of your body. You will want to take the calculations below:

- Bust: weigh your bust all the way around, holding the measuring tape in line with your nipples.
- Chest: weigh your breasts or pectoral muscles immediately below and all the way down your back.

- Waist: find the narrowest portion of your waist, usually just below your ribcage, and weigh it all around.
- Hips: find and weigh the largest position of your hips all the way around.
- Thighs: weigh the whole round of the upper leg, when standing straight.
- Knees: weigh just above the knee all the way around, when standing straight.
- Upper arms: weigh the whole proportion of your upper arms above the elbows.
- Lower arms: weigh the entire part of your lower arms under your elbows.

You will need a non-stretchable measuring tape to properly measure. Hold the amount of tape across the body, parallel to the surface. Wrap the tape across your body as close to your skin as possible when you are measuring your measurements, but don't pinch so closely that the tape measure cuts into your skin or creates an indentation. Getting someone else taking your measurements for you is good so you can stand straight; if you don't have someone at your side, take your measurements in front of a mirror and make sure you keep the tape steady and weigh in the correct spots.

Make a list of your measurements in a notebook or notepad for your phone. Take the measurements every couple of weeks and log the numbers every time at the same location. You can use the metrics to track your progress as time goes on.

Expect Ups And Downs

Like anything in life, with intermittent fasting you'll experience ups and downs, particularly at the very start. Don't expect all to go right off the bat perfectly and don't get lost in glory. You'll slip up: sometimes you'll snack outside your feeding slot, and that's all right. If you go into it knowing you're trying to put your best foot forward but still realizing it can take a little while to get used to the change, you're going to be less likely to beat yourself up when things don't go absolutely according to schedule.

CHAPTER 10.
Who Can Do Intermittent Fasting And Who Cannot

Who Should Fast?

As it happens, you don't need to be tangled in a problem before you have it all solved. So, even if you don't have real excess fats to burn, intermittent fasting is a good way to maintain your weight.

I advise young ladies to try intermittent fasting.

That's because it's a safe trick from sexual, marital and birth complications. It keeps your skin radiant, as I've told you while explaining autophagy.

I guess holy spirit already spoke to the high schoolers, they somehow made sure they never complete their diet. Ask the moms.

Married women and those with kids should try intermittent fasting too.

Especially those who notice that their bellies continue to bulge like a balloon even after giving birth.

Nothing is wrong with you medically, but your man married a flat portable lady, not a balloon bellied.

He may love you a lot alright, but don't give him a chance to think about other women he meets every day at work who have what you used to have.

I'm still going to discuss the chances of working women and intermittent fasting in full, just a few pages away.

So if you ask me, intermittent fasting is for all girls, ladies, women. As long as there's no health complication of any sort initially.

Who Shouldn't Fast?

Now what happens if you have a couple of health problems before?

I hate to tell you that it really may not be a brilliant idea to try out intermittent fasting. Although, the complexity determines your chances of trying intermittent fasting.

For instance, if it's some menstrual pain that stops with menstruations, and your monthly flow doesn't flow like you are a planning to fill a tank, you shouldn't have a problem trying intermittent fasting.

But you might face real issues if you usually have overflow of blood and you fast again.

If you are underweight, or you have been told that rather than lose some, you need more weight, I would cross out any chance of fasting if I were you.

If you are usually anxious too or your doctors are still trying to get you working on a healthy feeding style, the numerous benefits may be too attractive to leave, but your weight and focus must be on your body balance.

Some people think it's a bad idea to let kids fast.

Well, a young woman who hasn't started her menses may try intermittent fasting, just that there are chances her puberty could be delayed if she fasted for too long.

So, it's always advised that when your little chubby girl tries it, it is once in a while. Just once a few times and she'll be safe.

Apart from such kind of problems, if you are on a constant diet of some kind, or perhaps drugs and you might have to pause them to fast, it makes no sense to even hope to.

If you are a cancer, ulcer or one of the few other 'cers' patient, I think it makes sense to see your doctor before starting any diet plan.

Apart from these few conditions, we also need to talk about a couple other states, everyone can fast, except some I want to mention below.

A Woman On Menstruation.

As I guess you would be aware, that monthly blood that breaks from a woman's vagina and flows at regular times is called menstruation.

We know it goes on for a few days, sometimes 3, and 8 at most.

Does yours go longer than that?

That means you have to see a doctor urgently, before you even think of a diet table.

If yours is okay, then 'we can probably calculate your chances of fasting intermittently together', as Dr. Roberts would say.

Because menstruation can make you feel weak, you need your strength, your stamina, your meals and all calories you can get during your monthly flow. But fasting means your body gets only a few supplies.

If you are not planning a very long intermittent fasting period, and you live a very healthy life before, you shouldn't have any problem with fasting because there's this nutrient reserve inside you that your body turns to for help.

If that's not the case, intermittent fasting could mean that the part of your brain that coordinate your regular monthly flow called 'hypothalamus' will be too hungry to work, and gonadotropin releasing hormones (those ones see to your monthly flow in the ovaries) and the pituitary gland are affected too. what happens?

You bag irregular and disrupted menstrual cycle.

It can even get worse if you are on a long period intermittent fasting because your nutrient reserve will likely be too low to supply enough calories, and it can get to that point where your body system switches off your reproductive organs.

It says "hey, close that baby factory, this girl has got nothing to feed a baby, so just shut the doors, we open when she has enough nutrients to fund our business again'.

Of course, you can have sex but the eggs won't be formed.

The moment you supply enough nutrients, that body system returns to normal.

So, on mensuration, should you fast during intermittent fasting? Tell me, I'm all ears.

Pregnancy

Dear potbellied sister, I am going to be very frank with you right now.

You love something doesn't make it ideal for you. Intermittent fasting can really help your brain, burn your fats, help your cells reproduction and help your food digestion, yes, I know all of them.

But I am sorry to tell you, your pregnancy ends your fast, till delivery at least.

Why?

Because you've got a baby inside your stomach who doesn't bloody care about all those hellacious treatments you are finding yourself.

It needs you to have more weight, meaning more fats, more sugar and to eat any possible thing at any time they come like the biblical fish that ate everything, including Jonah.

So, fasting for a pregnant? Possible, just not ideal.

Breast-feeding

Now let's turn to the baby mothers.

Hey bouncing baby mother!

How are you?

Has your ballooned belly refused to deflate after delivery?

Have you tripled your size despite delivery and now you want me to tip you?

Forget the jokes, you are asking the right person.

It's okay to still have a very large tummy after birth. Or a kind of weight around that old size you had while pregnant.

It is okay, but if you can return to the former gracefully slender lady that everyone knew, why hold on to an old version?

Dr. Macron had often repeated that breast feeding women can practice intermittent fasting too. Most women were always fat in his own home after delivery.

So they mildly practiced intermittent fasting after delivery and they were fine. So, dear mother, it's a yes.

But I have to ring in it your head as we were taught, you need about 1800 calories to supply nutritious milk per day, how do you plan to supply that for over a year if you are not getting it yourself?

Well, if you are keeping it as mild as possible, say only 8-10 hours per day.

That's on a 10:14 fasting to eating ratio.

You are not likely to be affected, and you can gradually tackle all inflammation, you can even ensure autophagy that way.

So, if you must fast, strictly make it no longer than I said.

A Woman On Menopause

Hi granny!

We got your package too.

While it is very possible to reach menopause (that's when you don't menstruate anymore) at 47, the ideal age is about 58 upwards.

Your autophagy rate will likely reduce as you grow older, but becoming a grandma doesn't mean you have to suffer from excess insulin, calories fat, a dull brain, an unhealthy digestive system and inflammation among others, right?

Great, I really think you should try intermittent fasting.

There was this old and very grey haired woman among us who was always complaining because she was too fat and her legs would not take her oversized body anywhere.

I know she got a lot better after fasting, but she probably did it for a very long period which I don't recommend for old women. Short periods can cure you too.

Intermittent fasting can boost your immunity, your digestion, your brain functioning, your balance weight campaign and of course your general healthiness.

It's worth a trial really, but be careful, I don't want to be told you fasted for forty days, you are already too old to be Jesus.

So if you are among those I said can practice intermittent fasting, then be sure you do it moderately, don't toy with a baby's neural growth just because you want less fat, make it moderate.

But as people often ask me, if you are a very busy woman, does it make sense to try intermittent fasting?

CHAPTER 11.
Intermittent Fasting For Pregnant Women

It is not risk-free: Intermittent fasting is not advisable to people who are at higher health risks such as those over sixty-five years. People under medical conditions, high fat needs, the diabetic, the underweight, the underage, pregnant, and those breastfeeding cannot undertake intermittent fasting.

You will be hungry: During intermittent fasting, you might have a grumbling stomach, especially if you have correctly been observing the correct dietary plans. You should avoid looking at, smelling, or even thinking about food while fasting since this trigger the releasing o gastric acids in your stomach, which then makes you hungry. Engage in some other activities, but if you wish to fill your water, drink herbal tea or other drinks free from calories. You may note increased food intake in the non-eating days where you are not limited to any calorie intakes. Intermittent fasting triggers binge food consumption. There could also be cases of cravings, especially after increased levels of cortisol hormone.

Dehydration: Lack of eating may make you forget to take water. You might fail to take note of the thirst cues when fasting.

Fatigue: Intermittent fasting makes you feel tired, especially if you are trying it for the first time. Your body tends to run short of energy and disrupts your sleep patterns, and this comes along with a feeling of being tired.

Irritability: Since intermittent fasting helps in mood regulation, it can as well regulate your appetite. It leads to being depressed and upset.

Intermittent fasting long-term consequences are not known: Since no one knows whether after losing weight, you will maintain the same for some years, studies claim that no relevant evidence to support the extent of intermittent fasting. You are, therefore, always advised to talk to your doctor for sound advice on how you should practice intermittent fasting.

There are precautions that you should undertake when practicing intermittent fasting. Fasting has been there since time immemorial, and in some religions, it is considered as a holy practice. Whatever way, you may start practicing intermittent fasting; you should follow its essential tips to avoid any inconveniences. Therefore, you should:

Ensure that your body is fit for fasting. It is by making sure that you are not pregnant, not under any medication, no health complications, not underage, or even diabetic. If you cannot fast, then you can always change to cleaner eating habits such as eating natural foods and eliminate any sugar, rich, or fatty foods from your diet.

Before starting intermittent fasting, you should always try and consult your doctor. Your doctor will give updates about your health concerns and advise whether the step is necessary or not.

Try and make intermittent fasting fit into your lifestyle. You should never fast during the times you are stressed or under excess exertion. It is advisable if you are a newbie in intermittent fasting to try the 5:2 way of fasting whereby you can fast on the first day of the week, then on Thursdays so that you can prepare to take your favorite meals over the weekend.

Before you start intermittent fasting, do not gorge yourself with a 'last supper,' but you should instead take healthy meals, lean proteins, and vegetables. Fruits have natural sugar and including them in your meal could mean a lot. A little amount of starch could make the meal complete, as well. A meal that has all these nutrients will make your body survive the fasting period.

Prepare your household, body, and thoughts before starting intermittent fasting. It means that you should have enough rest and get prepared emotionally. Think about your aim and how to achieve it. Make sure that you hide or keep out of reach any foods that could tempt you during your fasting period.

Stop pretending to be a hero, even when your body is weak. Do not push your body too hard in the name of fasting. There are some of the symptoms that should be of great concern during your fasting time. You should take note of heart shudders, light-headedness, and general feebleness. It requires the use of common sense because you cannot force your body to do what it cannot.

Do not engage in tough exercises; do light ones. Engage in massages as they help have even blood flow in the body parts full of calories, thus reducing cortisol. Do not burn the muscles for energy while fasting.

Always take your vitamins depending on the method of fasting you choose. That acts as a supplement, especially if in liquid form, as it eases the process of digestion. They help compensate the vitamins lost while fasting.

Never forget to take a lot of water every fasting day. Your urine should alert you if it is not light in color. If not so, drink desirable amounts of water for proper hydration.

Since you are fasting, it is an obstacle to associating with your friends who are having fun, eating chocolates, and drinking wine since you will get tempted to take some. You can indulge in other ways of having fun with your friends. You can pay a visit to the nearest mall, window-shop new clothes or electronics. Avoid grocery stores and any dinner dates. Clear any mouth-watering photos from your gallery.

Avoid getting stressed since stress increases the levels of cortisol, which is responsible for fat storage and muscle breakdown. You can practice yoga, meditating, or having deep breaths. Your body needs enough energy to last you during the fasting period, and so these exercises should be light and not vigorous.

To avoid freaking out, you can always invite your friends to accompany you in doing intermittent fasting. The idea of creating your fasting thread or checking online for any other people doing intermittent fasting can help you master your progress. That is the time that you should focus on mentally cleaning your closet and reflecting on what you are doing.

Avoid 'Victory Binging.' Many people indulge themselves after the fasting period. You should take in a healthy meal and avoid foods that cannot get digested easily. You should take in foods rich in fiber, and if you are alcoholic, remember to take care when resuming.

CHAPTER 12.
A Proper Shopping List

A planned food guide for the first two weeks of intermittent fasting can help you with meal planning, shopping, and feel better psychologically.

The 16: 8 protocol is the best in these cases, to gradually begin to enter intermittent fasting with the right spirit, feel less uncomfortable and enjoy healthy food.

The best cuisine you can use is definitely the steamed one. Foods remain rich in the active ingredients of which they are made, without added fats and with the authentic taste of food. Minerals and vitamins are not wasted and remain entirely inside the vegetable.

I love the steam kitchen and it fits perfectly with a healthy and healthy lifestyle that involves less waste of time, of elaborate dishes, but that leaves taste and a good line.

Let's start using centrifuges, extractors or blenders. During the hours you can eat, two balanced meals will make you rediscover the desire to eat "well" and when you are hungry, without giving your body more, which is not desired and which, as we have seen, is only a source of undisputed healthy issues.

Smoothies, centrifuges or fruit and vegetable extracts will visibly improve your health and your life.

Daily use makes the skin brighter and provides those substances that our body needs, which are easy to remove and are not complex sugars that peep out in the rolls of fat.

Let's see together a weekly menu prepared for the first week:

Here is the simple recipe for a cream. You can use it replacing it with a meal or when you don't have a huge hunger. It's almost a late breakfast

Budwig Cream: these Budwig The ingredients of the cream, which Dr. Kousmine has created inspired in turn to the recipe of the German Dr. Budwig, known for research sue on acids fat:

- flax seed ground (1 tablespoon and a half)
- A freshly ground Other oil seeds (hazelnuts, almonds, walnuts, etc.).
- bananas (100 gr) or 1 teaspoon of honey
- a seasonal fruit (100 gr Cut into small pieces)
- lemon juice
- 1 tablespoon Whole grains finely ground
- Yogurt organic cow or soy (125gr) or tofu (75gr) or lean cottage cheese (100g) as an alternative if you like you can use cooked legumes

It can be salty, too: just ADD flax, oats, tomato (100g), a stick of celery, yogurt, scallions, a pinch of oppurelino sale, rice, a large carrot, parsley handful, lean cottage cheese, half an apple and little sales.

MONDAY

Meal 1: radish salad, rape and spinach. Mackerel baked with garlic and parsley (or hummus), rye bread, sour steamed artichokes

Meal 2: Belgian, arugula and radishes. Barley and beans spinach stews with olives and almonds

TUESDAY

Meal 1: arugula, radish and fennel rice with fresh asparagus beans cooked cabbage steamed with herbs

Meal 2: dandelion, Jerusalem artichokes and celeriac soup with vegetables (onions, carrots, spinach or chard, cabbage) with buckwheat and pinto

WEDNESDAY

Meal 1: carrots, raw champignons, artichokes 2 poached eggs with green sauce (parsley, garlic and capers) stewed potatoes and leeks

Meal 2: lettuce, turnips and radishes couscous with stewed peas and mixed vegetables (cabbage, carrot, celery, leek)

THURSDAY

1 Meal: Fennel, dandelion, shallots sardines with raisins and pine nuts (or marinated and grilled tofu) and cauliflower cream

Meal 2: Chinese cabbage Salad, loquats oats and spring onions and artichokes with mashed chickpeas

FRIDAY

1 Meal: Marinated cauliflower, carrots and artichoke polenta with rabbit stew (or with beans), stewed beets with garlic and chilli

Meal 2: Jerusalem artichoke salad, green radicchio and radishes rice and lentils, rape stewed with garlic and rosemary

SATURDAY

Meal 1: curly lettuce, cabbage, apple, radish rice with porcini mushrooms, chicken breast in mushroom sauce or baked omelette with mushroom sauce, cauliflower au gratin with vegetable sauce

Meal 2: pickled cabbage hood with raisins and almonds; Escarole and bulgur with orange lentils, stewed artichokes with garlic and herbs of Provence

SUNDAY

Meal 1: marinated pumpkin, fennel and artichokes roasted turkey with potatoes; Stewed onions with balsamic vinegar (for vegetarians: lasagna with lupins, marinated tofu kebabs)

Meal 2: salad of grated carrots with green sauce (garlic and parsley) Saraceno with soy cream and turmeric; stewed cabbage with tomato concentrate; laurel Beans

Now let's see some recipes, useful for your subsequent meals, based a lot on a diet rich in lipids and proteins and low in carbohydrates. We will also see centrifuge recipes, smoothies and fruit and vegetable extracts.

Juices And Smoothies Recipes

Centrifuge Detox

Ingredients:

1 celery leg
3 leaves of white cabbage
parsley
1 apple

Wash and dry the ingredients well by cutting them into small pieces and removing the apple core and skins for spinning. Put celery, white cabbage and the one apple into the centrifuge. Turns on. At the end, put parsley.

Green Extract..or Meal!

Ingredients:

Sicilian half broccoli
2 leaves of black cabbage
½ lime
½ lemon
1 kiwi
1 green pepper
1 green apple

Wash and clean the vegetables and fruit. Leave it in small pieces and insert it gradually into the juice extractor. Finally leave lemon and lime. Excellent juice, with rich properties of Vitamin C and an excellent detoxifying. Broccoli in particular has anti-tumor prevention properties (like all cruciferous ones). Satisfying even for an excellent meal replacement, adding dried fruit to accompany

Red Juice
Ingredients:

2 carats
1 lemon
1 beetroot

Wash dry and place in small pieces in the juice extractor. the turnip is an excellent anti-oxidant and contains nutrients for the microcirculation. Together with the carrots beta-carotene and the vitamin C of the lemon .. it is perfect for those who want to lose weight or lose cellulite

Juice of the day!
Ingredients:

1 banana
3 oz baby spinach
4 oz red cabbage
2 oz blueberries
2 oz endive salad

Wash vegetables and blueberries well and cut into small pieces. Place them in the extractor and prepare the juice. Excellent mineralizer, rich in vitamins and antioxidant

Strawberry Smoothie, Raspberries and Yogurt

Ingredients:

1 oz strawberry

1 oz raspberry

1 banana

2 white yogurt

Pour the yogurt and fruit in the blender. Work and make a thick cream. Enrich yourself with chopped almonds and walnuts, coconut. It is an excellent recipe rich in magnesium, fibers and proteins that helps intestines and serotonin on gray days.

Recipe For Your Health

A healthy and balanced diet, based on an intermittent fasting regime, helps not only to lose weight easily, but to give us those functional nutritional inputs for our body. This means less time spent in the gym, better nutrients, better health, improved chronic conditions and disorders or diseases such as: diabetes, PCOS (Polycystic Ovary Syndrome), Thyroid (Ipo and Hypothyroidism or Hashimoto's Thyroiditis), Arthritis, Endometriosis, Cardiovascular Disorders, Blood Pressure, Chronic Fatigue (a pathology in some states recognized as health-related), Fibromyalgia.

Let us remember that the role of insulin and hormones therefore, which are secreted from the body by the adrenal glands, play a very important role in our body and are often responsible for many ailments.

Magical Smoothie

Ingredients:

2 tablespoons flax seed meal
2 cups frozen spinach
2 tablespoons chia seeds
1 scoop whey protein
five cubes ice
3 cups water

Time: 10 minutes

Wash and cut all the ingredients into pieces, after which, place them in the blender. Mix and turns on. Then pour into 2 glasses and serve.

Cheese Waffles

Ingredients:

½ of cup Parmesan cheese, shredded
2 eggs
1 onion
1 cup of mozzarella cheese
½ teaspoon black pepper
1 cup cauliflower

Time: 20 minutes

Wash the vegetables.

Dry them. Place all the ingredients (excluding the eggs) in a blender and blend. Take the mixture and place it in a bowl. Mix everything and pour 1 ladleful, on a non-stick pan or in the electric waffle machine.

Salmon and Asparagus

Ingredients:

1 teaspoon EVO oil (olive)

4 asparagus stalks

2 salmon fillets

¼ cup butter

1 lime

salt

black pepper

Preheat the oven at 355 level. Wash the salmon and place it on a cloth to dry. Spice up its surface with peppercorns. Sprinkle with fresh lime and a pinch of coarse salt. Take the asparagus aside. Cook them in steam or in a little salted water for a few minutes. When half cooked, remove from the heat.

Take a baking dish. Spread the bottom with 1 teaspoon of oil. Put the salmon and asparagus. 2 flakes of butter over the salmon. Cook for 20 minutes. Remove from the oven and sprinkle with fresh lime again

Mushroom Pie

Ingredients:

1 cup of sliced mushrooms

1 cup baby spinach

6 diced bacon slices

10 egg

½ cup of crumbled goat cheese

olive oil

salt

black pepper

Time: 30 minutes

Preheat the oven to 180 degrees Celsius.

In a large oven pan, heat the oil and place over medium high heat. Sauté the mushrooms for 3 minutes and brown them lightly. Add the spinach and the bacon and sauté for 1 minute until the spinach is wilted. Then add the eggs and cook for 3 or 4 minutes lifting the edges of the "omelette" with a spatula. Body of crumbled cheese. Season with salt and pepper and then bake for about 15 minutes.

Pumpkin pie

Ingredients:

olive oil

500 g sausage

8 egg

2 cup of butternut pumpkin

1 tablespoons of fresh oregano

salt

black pepper

½ cup of cheddar cheese

Preheat the oven to 190 degrees Celsius. Grease a baking dish lightly with olive oil and set aside. In a large pan, heat olive oil over medium high heat. Brown the sausage for 5 minutes until cooked. While the sausage is on the fire, beat the eggs with the pumpkin and the oregano in a bowl. Season with salt and pepper. Add the cooked sausage and stir, then pour it into the pan. Sprinkle with cheese and cover it with aluminum foil. Bake for about 30 minutes, remove the sheet and then cook another 15 minutes.

CHAPTER 13.
Diet For Intermittent Fasting

Intermittent fasting lets you eat whenever you want and however you want. If you are dedicated to losing weight, then you should follow a proper diet. Though fasting techniques will help you to lose fat, you can increase the rate by eating foods that regulate the burning of the extra fat in your body.

Even if you decide to follow a meal plan for your diet, you will still have many things to eat during your non-fasting period. Whether you are following the 16/8, 5:2, 24-hour or alternate day method of IF, there are still times when you can eat what you like. However, you will get the most benefits from your weight-loss regime if you stick to certain foods at your breakfast, lunch and dinner times. To help you make the right choices, here are the items which you should eat at these times.

Breakfast

If you are following a fasting plan that allows you to have an early breakfast, then you should try consuming these foods.

Green Smoothie

The low sugar levels and healthy fats in it keep you satiated until lunch, and it is great for regulating digestion.

Preparation Method

Add avocado, chia seeds, coconut milk, and spinach to your blender and drink it up.

Mint Chip Protein Shake

It is full of protein, greens and wholesome ingredients.

Preparation Method

You just need to mix avocado, Greek yogurt, protein powder, mint/peppermint, milk, and spinach.

Egg Muffins

Eggs are a great source of proteins and important vitamins.

Preparation Method

All you would need for making delicious egg muffins are bell pepper, onions, tomatoes, eggs, some spinach, salt, and hot sauce.

Chocolate Coconut Protein Balls

These protein balls are satiating and keep you full for a long time.

Preparation Method

Mix coconut, oats, chocolate chips, honey, and some protein powder, and your healthy breakfast item is ready.

Oatmeal

The traditional breakfast for dieting people is oatmeal.

Preparation Method

Choose your flavor and just add some milk.

Hard-boiled or Scrambled Egg

The goodness of eggs is known by all. The vitamins and other nutrients present in an egg are good for your bones and muscles.

Lunch

This would be included in almost all meals during your fasting and non-fasting periods. Make it a nutritious meal with moderate calories and high satiation. The following items can help you achieve that.

Baked Potato

They give you steady energy and lasting fullness for a longer period. They are very high in carbohydrates, vitamins, and fibers.

Roasted Vegetables

Veggies are a ready-made source of all the nutrients that your body needs. A high amount of vegetables in a diet is very helpful in burning body fat.

Avocado Toast with Crushed Peanuts

This simple food item contains a lot of healthy fat and fiber. All you need to do is toast a slice of bread and spread the avocado onto it. You can add spices for your taste too.

Chicken, Vegetable or Bean Soup

Soups allow you to take in a maximum amount of nutrition. All the goodness of the ingredients that you add gets added up in the soup.

Avocado/Chicken/Vegetable Salad

Preparation method

Raw vegetables have more nutrition than roasted or fried ones. You can add dressings and spices of your choice to make a delicious salad. Including chicken, meat and avocado in your salad will increase the nutritional profile of your lunch.

Chickpea Salad

Chickpeas make a great replacement for meat in a vegetarian or vegan diet. They reduce the risk of several diseases, improve digestion and help in weight loss.

Tuna Pita Sandwiches

Tuna has amazing benefits for your body. Your tuna sandwich will be healthy if you do not dress it up with mayonnaise and baked bread.

Broccoli Slaw Salad

Boiled broccoli prevents many diseases. A person wanting to lose weight must have broccoli on his/her shopping list.

Dinner

The final meal of the day should be light yet fulfilling. It should boost metabolism and increase the digestion since you will not be eating until the next day. Meals that you can use for your meal plan are given below.

Spicy Chicken Chili

Spices, chicken, and chili peppers are all good for your body. They help in losing weight and increasing muscles and metabolism. They form a very enriching and fulfilling dinner.

Quinoa Salad

Quinoa is one of the healthiest and most nutritious foods that exist. It is rich in fibers, protein and amino acids, which are great for weight loss.

Shrimp Fried Rice

This low-fat food contains fibers and proteins. It makes a very healthy yet tasty choice for dinner. Vegetarians and vegans can add broccoli and soybeans instead of shrimp to their fried rice.

Lemon Garlic Chicken Drumsticks

Lemon, garlic, and chicken boost your metabolism and clear the stored waste inside the body.

Seafood

Fish, salmon, anchovies, tuna, and char are all rich in omega-3 fatty acids. They are great for your heart, brain, and bones.

Roasted Vegetables

They can be a part of your lunch and dinner alike, based on your mood, IF plan and taste.

Steak

Steak is loaded with protein and is good for your waistline. Make sure you get lean cuts of this red meat to keep the calorie intake low.

Snack Time

There are times between the big meals when your stomach craves food. Satisfy your hunger by eating food that is light and low in calories. Go for these healthy snacks when you crave food between your meals. Each of them is high in nutritional value and will help you to feel full for a longer time.

Fruit of Choice (Apple, Banana, Berries)
Almonds
Protein Bar
Yogurt
Edamame
Carrots
Zucchini Chips
Cottage Cheese
Low-Sugar Ice Cream
Lemon juice

Meal Plan

There are seven days in a week, and you have already been provided with more than seven options for each of your meals. You can now make your meal plan according to your liking and taste. Choose the meals that you would prefer, design your 7-day plan, and stick to it to achieve maximum weight loss.

CHAPTER 14.
Fasting For Women Over 50

Overweight women over 50 have a higher risk of diabetes and heart problems than they did when they were younger. IF is one option they have to manage their weight and control these health risks.

The metabolism of a woman over 50 has become slower, so you can't expect quick results if you are a member of this group, but you will probably get the most out of it than any other group of women because of all the anti-aging effects of IF and autophagy.

Overweight and obese people have higher risks of heart disease, stroke, and more as they age. On the other hand, thinner people are not looking at these same risks.

Losing weight can only be good for your body, and autophagy is the healthiest and most effective way to do it. Autophagy will help you stay thin, feel good, and be healthy for years and years.

But, so far, we have only talked about the health benefits that are immediately obvious. There is also a reduction of health risks that are not cosmetic like youthful skin and weight loss. It has been proven that an increase in autophagy reduces your risk of Alzheimer's and Parkinson's disease.

More autophagy also reduces inflammation, which will increase your overall health. There has even been research about the benefits of autophagy for cancer patients undergoing chemotherapy.

Studies have shown that cancer patients going through chemotherapy saw a reduction in the clumps of white blood cells that accumulate because of chemotherapy. Dead cells can be hazardous to your body if they are not cleaned out during autophagy.

Since these patients fasted in order to turn on autophagy, their bodies were able to clean out the white blood cells and recover from chemotherapy sooner.

You can only imagine the kind of advantage you get if you are turning autophagy on as much as possible, and you aren't even looking at a major health risk yet. You may not have as big an accumulation of dead cells as someone going through chemotherapy, but if you have not fasted before and you don't exercise regularly, it is very likely that you have a lot of toxins in your body.

This is because if you don't go through autophagy very often, materials like dead cells, dead organelles, and unused proteins start to pile up and make your cells less efficient.

Putting your body through autophagy doesn't just combat aging in ways that are immediately visible. It also greatly reduces your risk of long-term age-related disease. Whether you're looking to improve the quality of your life or the length of your life, making autophagy happen in your body will do it.

There are many misconceptions about how autophagy does its anti-aging work. Perhaps the most common is that its only health benefits come from taking care of toxins. Clearing toxins from your system is certainly a good thing, but autophagy goes far beyond ridding your body of harmful chemicals.

Most of these toxins are not from outside your body, but they are materials like proteins and organelles that your cells used once and then no longer had a use for. These discarded materials start to take up space over time, creating clutter that slows down your cells. This is when they become toxins.

Some of these toxins cause even worse problems than congestion. The worst case is protein clusters that form in the brain. Neurodegenerative diseases like Alzheimer's become more of a concern as we age, and autophagy might be your best ally in fighting against your risk of these diseases.

From a broader perspective, Alzheimer's manifests as "knots" and "tangles" in the brain that impair memory.

When doctors look at the knots and tangles with a microscope, they see that these irregularities are actually clusters of proteins that have built up over time. They are proteins that brain cells used at one point but later had no purpose. The protein clusters were not managed with autophagy, so they simply accumulated and started leading to serious memory problems.

Alzheimer's disease is the most extreme consequence that you can have from not going through enough autophagy. It is not the only consequence, however. Discarded materials like protein clusters start to build up throughout your body if you rarely go through autophagy.

In this regard, low autophagy leads to a low count of collagen, the protein that makes your skin youthful. Your skin cells can't produce collagen when they are crowded by cellular garbage.

Similarly, you lose more muscle mass if you rarely go through autophagy because you are not turning on autophagy to repair the muscle tissue damage that results from physical activity.

From these examples alone, you can see that autophagy is more than a toxin-cleaning agent. Autophagy doesn't only destroy the bad (toxins); it builds the good (new organelles, proteins, and cells). Both sides of autophagy make it such a powerful anti-aging tool, one that was surprisingly given to us by nature.

So far, we have established that autophagy isn't just good for destroying pathogen invaders — it also destroys materials that become toxic when they linger in the cell for too long. In short, this biological process cleans out toxins from the outside and inside.

In the third stage, your cells use these broken-down parts as ingredients to build new cells and cell structures. What's more: your cells have more room to build new cells and new cell parts because they freed up so much space during autophagy.

All these things come together when you find a way to turn on autophagy on a regular basis. Equipped with all this information, you know much more about autophagy than even your average fasting practitioner.

Women over 50 certainly still want to manage their weight and have good skin, but it is around this age that we start to get a more mature perspective on life, and we care more about the health consequences of our daily life choices than before. They have many options for unlocking autophagy even further than they would with IF alone.

Back in the 90s, the idea of caloric restriction became very popular, and people saw improvements in their health from doing nothing more than eating less. There is even a great deal of evidence that mammals who restrict their calories live longer than mammals who do not.

This has not yet been proven to be true for humans, but still, restricting your caloric intake can only be a good thing. You get this additional benefit from turning on autophagy through fasting while also getting the benefit of autophagy itself along with it.

We have heard a lot of ideas about losing weight from nutritionists in the last few decades, but let's not kid ourselves: the main reason for weight gain across the planet comes down to people consuming a lot of calories without physically exerting themselves to burn them off. Fasting for any length of time will lead to consuming fewer calories, so you are on the right track for losing weight when you fast.

The next popular method of turning on autophagy is the keto diet. This method will turn on autophagy because it involves depriving your body of nutrients that it would normally consume for energy.

However, following the keto diet alone will not turn on autophagy because it is only activated when your cells are in a state of stress, and as long as you are sedentary or filling your body with any kind of food, your cells are not in this state.

That said, since the keto diet is so low in carbs, this style of eating will aid in turning on autophagy. I definitely recommend following the keto diet because the mistake many autophagy practitioners make is consuming a lot of carbs while they are not fasting.

Eating a lot of carbs will prevent your body from fasting for a long time because it takes a long time for your digestive system to process them. Not only that, but as you may be aware, it becomes harder to keep weight off the older you get, and you are significantly slowing down the process of burning fat when your digestive tract has a backlog of carbs. Fighting against this problem is the role of the keto diet in anti-aging and autophagy.

Next, there is the method of good old exercise. Studies have shown that resistance training, also known as strength training, is the most effective way of turning on autophagy, saying it is even more effective than fasting. The reason for this is that when you use your muscles, you are getting tiny tears in your muscle tissue that are repaired through autophagy.

The unfortunate thing is that exercising might be the last thing that people want to do, even though it is so good for their health. Like the other methods, exercise has its own health benefits that are separate from autophagy.

Plenty of studies show that people who work out regularly have lower risks of all age-related illnesses, even those not related to the heart. If we are being honest, exercising is probably the best way to fight aging.

If you want to get the most out of autophagy, you should employ all of these methods together. When combined, the keto diet, exercise, and fasting will give you the greatest benefits, both in terms of weight loss and in general health.

If you don't yet feel motivated to be as healthy as possible, try to think of the autophagy in your cells as an analogy for your personal health. If they did not recycle their cellular garbage, your cells would simply die after their organelles stopped working or they were overcrowded with protein clusters and foreign invaders.

If you do not recycle your body's toxins by turning on autophagy regularly, your body will be over-encumbered with cellular garbage and you will be less healthy as a result. If this analogy were expanded, you might even live a shorter life if you do not regularly clean out your cellular garbage via autophagy.

Your cells try to live longer by using autophagy to combat their cellular aging — you should try to use autophagy to work against aging too.

CHAPTER 15.
How To Implement With Keto Diet

By now, you've probably heard of the Ketogenic Diet, nicknamed the Keto Diet for short. This is a very powerful and some say life-changing eating plan. It has some restrictions, so I only recommend it for those women who have really gotten comfortable with your Intermittent Fasting eating windows, eating healthier, and adding your own exercise regimen.

But once you have, then get ready for some miraculous body transformations. The Keto Diet is a diet of extremes. We're going to take the 'balanced diet' idea and completely throw it out!

The Keto Diet is a very high (good) fat, very low carb eating plan. We're talking over 100 grams of fat and less than 30 grams of carbohydrates per day. But it's these kinds of extremes that will get you massive results.

All About Ketosis

The Keto Diet actually changes your body's metabolic processes from one that mostly runs on glucose and glycogen from carbohydrates to one that primarily runs on ketones that come from those fat cells processed in your liver. When you are using ketones as your number one fuel, you're said to be in ketosis.

Take a look at the whole process in action:

You Eat Good Fats

Fats Enter the Stomach

Liver Breaks Down Fats For Energy (Beta-Oxidation)

Liver Produces Ketones

Ketones Used As Fuel

Liver Also Uses Stored Fat to Make Ketones

Ketones Used As Fuel

Say, look at that! We're back to using your stored fat as fuel, which is exactly what we want. You want to be in a state of ketosis while you're Intermittently Fasting in order to gain the maximum benefits from both.

How can you tell you're in ketosis? You will need to purchase a special monitor that can test your urine, breath, or blood to be sure. Your reading tells you exactly how many ketones your liver is producing for fuel. These monitors can be purchased online or at a store like Amazon or Walmart.

When you're just starting out on the diet, check for ketosis every day. Once you are in ketosis and you get a feel for that metabolic state in your body, then you can measure your ketones every three or four days. If you eat too many carbohydrate foods, you could knock yourself out of ketosis.

The Keto Macros

ecause in the Keto Diet world, those three are called Macronutrients. These 'Macros' form the basis for the Keto Diet and are the main thing you track each and every day. On the Keto Diet, calories matter, but not as much as getting the right amount of your Macros.

But your Macros on a Ketogenic Diet are vastly different.

You should be consuming 70% of your daily calories from those good fat sources, 19% of your proteins from natural animal and plant sources, and 5% - 8% of your carbohydrates from healthy sources.

For a woman's Macro requirements, it looks like this:

70% FATS – 19% PROTEINS – 5% CARBOHYDRATES

These are the Macros that you should track, and the proper percentages that you need in order to get into ketosis and stay in that metabolic state.

There are many online Ketogenic Macro calculators, and I encourage you to calculate your exact Macro percentages. They change depending on many factors in your physicality, including your height, weight, current age, and BMI.

As a general guideline when reading about the contents of these Macros on a food label, you should look for these quantities:

167g FATS – 100g PROTEINS – 25g CARBOHYDRATES

That adds up to 292 total grams of food per day. These are the Macros that you should be tracking each day that you're on the Ketogenic Diet.

These are the daily amounts that will kick your body into a ketosis state and start burning massive amounts of stored fat.

Keto Approved Foods

How are you supposed to eat nearly 170 grams of fat per day and yet far less than 30 grams of carbohydrates per day?

By sticking to the Keto Diet approved foods list! Below, I've put together the top 10 most common Ketogenic approved foods. This is an excellent base to get you started on the road towards changing your diet to the Keto one.

Produce:

~Avocados
~Lemons
~Onions
~Green Bell Peppers
~Button Mushrooms
~Romaine Lettuce
~Fresh Spinach
~Kale
~Broccoli
~Cauliflower

Meat & Seafood:

- ~Steak (Flank and Skirt)
- ~Ground Beef
- ~Bacon
- ~Shrimp
- ~Cod Fillets
- ~Boneless Chicken Breasts / Thighs
- ~Pork Chops
- ~Salami
- ~Prosciutto
- ~Lamb

Eggs & Dairy:

- ~Eggs
- ~High Quality Grass-Fed Butter
- ~Heavy Cream
- ~Cheddar Cheese
- ~Mozzarella Cheese
- ~Parmesan Cheese
- ~Cream Cheese
- ~Sour Cream
- ~Goat Cheese
- ~Plain Greek Yogurt

Herbs & Spices:

- ~Salt
- ~Pepper
- ~Fresh Garlic Cloves
- ~Fresh Herbs (parsley, cilantro, dill, etc.)

- ~Dried Italian Herbs
- ~Cinnamon
- ~Thyme
- ~Chili Powder
- ~Onion Powder
- ~Ginger

Oils & Condiments:

- ~Olive Oil
- ~Coconut Oil
- ~Sesame Oil
- ~Flavored Oils
- ~Mayonnaise
- ~Dijon Mustard
- ~Fish Sauce
- ~Hot Sauce
- ~Lemon Juice
- ~Soy Sauce

Nuts & Seeds:

- ~Macadamia Nuts
- ~Pecans
- ~Walnuts
- ~Almonds
- ~Nut Butters
- ~Pumpkin Seeds
- ~Sunflower Seeds
- ~Sesame Seeds

~Ground Flax Seeds

~Chia Seeds

Baking & Broths:

~Almond Flour

~Coconut Flour

~Cocoa Powder

~Baking Powder

~Vanilla Extract

~Sugar-Free Dark Chocolate

~Stevia

~Unsweetened Almond Milk

~Chicken Broth

~Beef Broth

Other:

~MCT Oil

~Green Olives

~Black Coffee

~Black or Green Teas

~Wine

~Dill Pickles

~Canned Tomatoes

~Full Fat Coconut Milk

~Curry Pastes (red, green, yellow)

~Psyllium Husk Powder

Those are the most essential eighty ingredients! There's plenty here to get you started. If you're having trouble meeting such a high fat requirement throughout your eating window, then take a look at the following foods and their high fat percentages:

~Butter – 100% fat

~Olive Oil – 100% fat

~MCT Oil – 100% fat

~Heavy Cream – 95% fat

~Green Olives – 88% fat

~Macadamia Nuts – 88% fat

~Cream Cheese – 88% fat

~Sour Cream – 86% fat

~Coconut Cream – 86% fat

~Walnuts – 84% fat

~Brazil Nuts – 84% fat

~Almond Butter – 79% fat

~Avocado – 77% fat

All of these foods are not only delicious, they can help you meet those fat gram requirements.

When you're on the Keto Diet, it's largely about the numbers. Eat as many good fats as you can to hit that high level required, keep your healthy protein intake to a medium level, and slash that carbohydrate number down to one that is very small.

If you have any questions about putting together meals from these ingredients and finding even more ingredients that are Keto approved,

I suggest you buy a specific Keto book! That will go into so much more detail.

The Keto Diet And Intermittent Fasting

Why do Intermittent Fasting and the Keto Diet work so well together?

That's because Intermittent Fasting helps your body get into ketosis faster and helps maintain that metabolic state even longer than if you weren't fasting.

What this means, is that you can supercharge the benefits that you get from Intermittent Fasting. You will go into ketosis quickly, and also begin burning the fat from your cells that much sooner.

Going Keto is the ultimate boost up for Intermittent Fasting.

CHAPTER 16.
16 The Science Of Intermittent Fasting

The human body has two main settings that determine how efficient, powerfully and smoothly our internal systems run. They help to boost energy throughout the day and provide extra fuel from stored fat cells to injured areas to help speed the healing process.

#1 Store Fat for Later Use: When people consume carbohydrates, sugars, and excess protein, the body digests it and uses it for the energy and nutrition it needs now, then transfers the remainder to the liver where it is converted into glycogen to be stored in fat deposits around the body in case of emergency. This is the process most active in the human body during feeding or feasting windows when food is being consumed regularly. When humans eat, the insulin production levels of the body increase thanks to the consumed sugars being digested and deposited in the liver as fat cells. When the liver itself can't hold any more fat but the human continues to eat, all new fat created from ingested food travels to other storage areas such as the core and thighs.

#2 Burn Stored Fat for Extra Fuel: This process is the one most active in times of fasting. Instead of relying on glucose delivered from food sources, the body is able to call upon stored fat cells to convert into emergency energy for the internal organs or body processes. This is the body's natural survival defense against starvation and can happen in times of distress such as being lost or at the mercy of harsh weather. It is also a process that can be initiated and controlled without risk of fatality or illness with Intermittent Fasting. It is monitored and upheld by a person's fluctuating glucose levels. When this begins, the body switches from running on empty sugar cells to burning excess fat so it can maintain energy until individual eats again.

Intermittent Fasting works by creating (and sticking to) a fasting schedule designed to control when the body slips in and out of these processes to minimize fat storage and maximize fat burning.

Intermittent Fasting For Cancer Prevention

Intermittent fasting reduces the development and progression of tumors in animal experiments. Rats on IF transplanted with a cancer cell line survived longer than free-fed animals. After 10 days, 50% of the IF animals were still alive compared to 12.5% in the control group.

Alternating fasting used only in middle age reduced the incidence of lymphoma in mice. In a 4-month observation period, 30% of the control mice became ill while none of the animals on intermittent fasting became cancerous. The researchers also found a better antioxidant activity, resulting in less development of harmful free radicals within the mitochondria (cell power plants). The antitumor effect did not result from the calorie reduction since both groups consumed the same amount of calories.

In rats, intermittent fasting reduced the development of pre-neoplastic (precursor to cancer) liver injury and liver nodules caused by a carcinogenic substance.

Unfortunately, human studies do not exist so far.

Lowered Cardiovascular Risk

In one study, intermittent fasting in non-obese participants resulted in an increase in good HDL cholesterol in women and a reduction in triglyceride levels in men. This effect occurred over 22 days in which every two days fasted. This change may have been caused by the degradation of body fat, which was -4%.

In the case of obese people, the values improved more clearly by an average weight loss of -5.6 kg after eight weeks of alternating fasting.

Total cholesterol dropped by 21%, LDL cholesterol by 25% and triglycerides by 32% while HDL cholesterol remained unchanged.

The systolic blood pressure dropped from 124 to 116 mmHg.

Stress resistance induced by intermittent fasting has a cardio protective effect beyond reducing body weight. Studies in mice show that in a heart attack, the affected tissue in the heart is half-smaller in alternately fasting mice than in normally fed animals. Also, in cardiac infarction, 4 times fewer cardiocytes die (heart muscle cells), when the animals were fed intermittently.

Calorie Independent Effect

Calorie restriction can have a positive effect on health and life expectancy. Some intermittent fasting researchers and advocates claim that starvation is more important than actually reducing calorie intake. Because fasting is a kind of stress for the body, it could stimulate the expression of genes that perform protective tasks and theoretically bring health benefits.

Some nutritionists assume that our ancestors did not consistently have food supplies, but were instead exposed to hunger periods and periods of increased caloric intake and those there genes were shaped and adapted accordingly. Thus, an alternate availability of food would be "natural."

IF partially dissociates the positive effect of calorie reduction from the actual total intake of calories. In mice, intermittent fasting results in improved glucose control, lower insulin levels, and greater resistance to neuronal damage regardless of weight loss or calorie intake.

Even without a reduction in calories, intermittent fasting increases the concentration of the hormone adiponectin. Adiponectin increases fat burning, anti-inflammatory, and antidiabetic and has a positive influence on cardiovascular health.

Distribution of fat deposits

In mice, intermittent fasting even without a weight loss leads to a redistribution of fat deposits in the body. The fat shifts from the visceral (in the abdomen) to the subcutaneous (under the skin) body fat. This change is healthier because visceral body fat is associated with increased inflammatory levels, insulin resistance, and metabolic syndrome. Although advocates often mention this effect of intermittent fasting, clinical studies have so far failed to detect a particularly increased decrease in visceral adipose tissue in humans.

Unfortunately, most versions of intermittent fasting, such as Eat Stop Eat, do not give users a healthy dietary change. The existing eating habits and the choice of food to be maintained, the method should only be a simplification to facilitate the calorie abstinence, however, a relearning is not promoted, which makes it easy to relapse into old habits, especially in obese people. There is a risk of migration between extremes: on the one hand fasting and on the other hand food cravings paired with the choice of low-nutrient and low-fiber, but high-calorie diet.

On the other hand, intermittent fasting provides a straightforward way to lose weight and, like any other diet, works better in some people than in others, depending on preference.

Fasting over 24 hours due to calorie restriction in calorie intake overshadows the negative effects on circadian rhythms caused by intermittent fasting, which merely shifts the meal timeslots towards evening (especially warrior diet, lean gains in part).

Side Effects

Intermittent fasting is usually very well tolerated, for some users the first few days on which they starve for longer are unusual and can cause irritation, fatigue or euphoria.

A double-blind, placebo-controlled, two-day study in which participants did not know if they were receiving any caloric or calorie-free food (in gel form) could not identify any side effects related to mental performance, physical activity, sleep, and whim.

A 24-hour Lent, without excessive exercise, lowers glycogen storage in the liver by almost 60%, so that the stored carbohydrates can easily maintain the blood sugar at a sufficient level. After 24 hours of fasting, the blood sugar level does not reach a pathological level (hypoglycemia). Also, the body can at any time through the process of gluconeogenesis produce sugar from amino acids and rely on ketones as a source of energy for the nervous system. However, this is unlikely as muscle breakdown in intermittent fasting is lower than in other diets, suggesting a muscle-sparing effect.

Diabetes 2 Risk

Humane studies have so far only observed a positive change in diabetes 2-related factors in men. Intermittent fasting increased insulin-mediated glucose uptake after 2 weeks, suggesting improved insulin sensitivity. These results are supported by another study in which male participants release less insulin after a 3-week alternating fast (always 36-hour fasting) in response to a meal, another indication of increased insulin sensitivity and thus a reduction in the risk of diabetes 2 Intermittent fasting, Women, on the other hand, developed inferior glucose tolerance during the same treatment because they had elevated blood sugar levels after a test meal.

At this point, it is essential to consider the small number of participants in the respective studies who can by no means provide definitive answers.

Aging Process

The restriction of calorie intake (calorie restriction, CR) is one of the most reliable methods to increase the lifespan of animals in animal studies significantly. Calorie restriction generally means a 10-30% daily reduction in daily caloric intake, resulting in an increase in the life span of various organisms from yeast, worms to nonhuman primates.

Calorie restriction is associated with improved insulin sensitivity, lowering of heart rate and blood pressure (which benefits cardiovascular health), reduced free radical damage to cellular components (proteins, DNA), reduced incidence of spontaneous and induced tumors and better resistance of neurons degenerative changes.

Intermittent fasting is an alternative to daily calorie restriction, with a similar effect on the aging process and lifespan. Alternating fasting in mice resulted in an extension of the average lifespan by 2.8-6.7 months when fasting was introduced at a young age. Several theories try to explain life-prolonging and health effects. Among other things, the stress caused by the calorie withdrawal could cause an overreaction of defense mechanisms, which allow the cells better defense against metabolic, genotoxic and oxidative stress, Intermittent fasting may be similar in effect to caloric restriction, but may be different, as the stress caused by starvation is more intense.

Brain Power and Aging

Both calorie restriction and intermittent fasting affect neuronal functionality, which decreases with age.

With advancing age, the so-called spine processes, which are located at the dendrites (branched cell processes) of neurons (nerve cells), decrease. The spine processes play an important role in the information transfer between the nerve cells. In rats, the number of thorns decreased by 38% after 24 months of a normal diet.

Intermittent fasting prevented the reduction of the density of the spine so that rats showed little difference to 6-month-old rats even after 24 months.

Calorie reduction by the intermittent fasting increased neurogenesis (formation of new brain cells), protected the neurons from dying and stimulated the production of BDNF (brain-derived neurotrophic factor), a protein associated with increased neurogenesis, in this way, if counteracts the deterioration of the aging process and improves the learning ability of older mice.

The effect on neurogenesis also appears to promote healing and functional recovery of spinal cord injuries in animals, whether intermittent fasting was introduced before or shortly after injury.

CHAPTER 17.
Everything You Need To Know About The Eat Stop Eat Program

Can You Fast For 24 Hours?

The Eat Stop Eat is not a daily fasting program, in fact, it mostly encourages you to fast just once per week. The fasting period, in this case, would be just 24 hours, which might sound a bit scary for some of you out there, but hear me out! How about if you had just one whole day of fast per week, and the rest of the week you can regularly? Can you cope with this program? The 24 hour fast is one of the most popular programs practiced by different people worldwide. It was developed by Brad Pilon who had the bright idea to name this program very simple: Eat Stop Eat.

There are plenty of specialists and people who can agree that this program is the easiest one, and perhaps it should be the first Intermittent Fasting program to be tried by beginners. Some people might be thinking of trying more IF programs, but you need to ease into Intermittent Fasting; to take it slow because you will be able to deal a lot easier with possible symptoms like hunger, headaches, and dizziness.

The Eat Stop Eat program is perhaps the most accessible and popular method for most Intermittent Fasting enthusiasts. Some people just like to fast completely for one day per week, every once in a while. Others are more ambitious and might want to try the 24 hours fast twice or three times a week. After all, it all depends on what you are looking to achieve. The beauty of this program is that it doesn't require any scheduling or special rules. You only have one rule: choose the day you want to fast! That's it!

Just like any other Intermittent Fasting program, this one doesn't mention anything about a special meal plan, you can eat whatever you want, as long as you respect the only rule that you have. Let's say that you like to hang out with your friends or family during weekends, have copious meals, and then you just want to fit in your favorite pair of jeans. In this case, I would strongly recommend having the fasting day on Tuesday or Wednesday, as you might not be able to have it on Monday (you are used to so much food during the weekend, so completely eliminating the food on Monday may be a bit too radical).

However, if you plan to try this program (or any Intermittent Fasting), you might need to take it easy with the calorie intake, as you probably want to lose some weight, or even to experience some other health benefits of Intermittent Fasting.

Is Cutting Down On Carbs Your New Meal Philosophy?

Sometimes, I wonder what is more dangerous to our bodies? Is it drugs, alcohol, tobacco? Well, I'm inclined to say that carbs are the most nocive to our bodies, especially that specific sub-group we also know as sugar. In some countries, there are extra fees for added sugar, so many drinks or products with excessive amounts of sugar cost more. By the way, have you looked recently at a bottle of Coca-Cola (or Pepsi), to see how much sugar it has? If not, then you might want to know that around 40% of the ingredients in those drinks is sugar.

This might make you think again about drinking (or giving to your children) any sodas, energy drinks, or normal natural juices (most of them have additional sugar, so it's not just fresh-squeezed juice). It's really hard to think that natural juice can only expire in a few months and no preservatives or special chemicals were added. Truth be told, every food or drink that is industrially processed can contain a high percentage of carbs. Even food that we consider normal can have a very high concentration of carbs. They can be found in bread, pastries, pasta, potatoes, rice, and many other products that are highly processed.

Pizzas or any other form of junk food have abundant carbs, so you might want to think again when eating all this food type. The problem with this food is that it has a very high-calorie level, but an extremely low nutrient value. Having just a burger with a soda next to eat is simply a caloric bomb, but guess what? You will feel hungry again in a short period; perhaps in less than 3 hours.

Sound familiar? Unfortunately, this type of food causes addiction, so as soon as you start feeling hungry again, your body will be craving for more carbs. Intermittent Fasting can help you control your calorie intake, but you need to make every calorie count, as you can't stuff your face with processed or junk food and expect to have results. Therefore, you need to be very careful with your nutrition, and cutting down on carbs should be your starting point. You need to find out what food you need to avoid or to minimize the consumption of it.

Therefore, this is what I'm suggesting: Try to eliminate the consumption of bread, pastry, and pasta (as much as possible)! Sorry, no sandwiches for you! Stay away from any fast-food place, and start eating more vegetables and fruits. You don't have to become vegan, but you need to carefully select the food you eat. Choose your own meal plan that best works for you!

If you don't have any idea about what you need to eat, try the Keto or the Mediterranean Diet! Since Intermittent Fasting is designed to make your body run on fats, basically making it the default "fuel," it's really important to keep eating fats. Now you are probably wondering: "But wait a minute! How can I eat fats and get slim?" Answering this question is really not complicated, as you stay away from glucose and carbs and keep fueling your body with fats to burn.

Remember, Intermittent Fasting means also a lower calorie intake, so basically the fats you are eating should never have the chance to get stored in your fat tissue. Nutrition plays a very important role in the success of any IF program, so this one should make no exception. You can have a few normal days of eating, but try to make them matter and eat a lot healthier, and focus on having LCHF (Low Carbs High Fats) meal plans.

How To Exercise During The Eat Stop Eat Program?

One of the best advantages of the 24 hours fast, is that you have plenty of feeding days; so, in other words, your body will not lack any macronutrients to function properly and to be energized. Like all the other Intermittent Fasting programs, the best way to work out is on an empty stomach. Some people would prefer just a few exercises to be in shape (like ab crunches or push-ups), whilst others prefer to jog, swim or to work out at the gym early in the morning.

In other words, you still need to enter the fasted state (on a daily basis) to find the best time for working out. So why not have a ten-hour eating period? Let's say from 9 am to 7 pm. This doesn't sound too harsh, does it? You can still have 3 main meals per day, and you can also enter the fasted state to workout on a daily basis, immediately after 7 am. For instance, if you have your last meal at 7 pm, you can head over to the gym early in the morning, and start training after 7 am. Usually, a normal training session should not last longer than 75 minutes, so this can give you plenty of time to have a shower, have a consistent breakfast (after 9 am) and get to work.

But what about the fast day? Can you workout during that day? As a matter of fact, it's highly recommendable to workout during that day. Training can give you the energy boost you need for the day, plus you will feel a lot better and more agile, as you will not feel the fat tissue slowing you down (at least not like it used to).

When you are on this program, it's better to find a way to work all of your muscle groups. Jogging can be a great way to burn calories, but it will not train all your muscles. However, swimming does, and you have plenty of equipment at your local gym to work out all the muscles of your body. Swimming can be a very pleasant way to get a lean body that you've always wanted, but if you want to increase in size and build muscles, you will also need to work out at the gym.

There is probably no need to point out to you the importance of breathing during a physical exercise, but it's still necessary to find out the best way to work out at the gym. When you are there, you need to be "beast" and train hard, so make every minute count. You are not there to sit and play on your phone, so you need to pull yourself together, find the inner motivation you need and don't waste time there. Therefore, I wouldn't encourage too long pauses between your exercises.

There are plenty of specialists who encourage the HIIT (High-Intensity Interval Training) method, as the best training you can have during your gym sessions. This method consists in having extremely intense exercises, for 20 seconds, followed by 10 seconds of rest, then repeat the session again, until you have eight complete sessions; so the exercise should last 4 minutes precisely. This is just an exercise, but you need to work out more muscles, so you need to have more exercise. Overall, the whole HIIT training session should be around 30 minutes.

Getting warmed up for such a session is highly important, so you need to have a few minutes of exercising the muscle groups you will train during the HIIT session. Cardio may be good for you, that's why there are so many people trying it, as a "prelude" to their workout. Regardless of your ambition when you work out, it's important to spend your time efficiently at the gym, otherwise, you are paying for your membership in vain.

You can have just one day of fasting per week if you work out on a daily basis in the fasted state, but if you want to maximize the results of this program, it's better to have 2 or even 3 fasting days per week.

Plus, if you have in the feeding period an LCHF meal plan, chances are that this Intermittent Fasting program will have amazing results.

CONCLUSION

Fasting: In ancient times, physicians used to cure certain diseases by interfering with their patient's meals. Epilepsy was considered as a supernatural disease in its origin as well as sure, and there was a proposal that nutritional treatment had a physical foundation. Some physicians claimed a possible cure of epilepsy as soon as it appeared through skipping of meals. The very first observation carried out in France in 1911, explaining that fasting was functional medicine for anyone with epilepsy was successful. The study involved 20 epilepsy patients and was of different ages. They were fed with foods with low fats, veggie diets, practiced together with some reasonable periods of fasting. Any epilepsy patient was to starve so that the disease can get cured. Fasting got popularized as a better method of restoring people's health. Many physicians recommended fasting for at least eighteen to twenty-five days to cure epilepsy. With a 90 percent water intake during the fasting period, many children and even young adults got cured of the epilepsy seizures. Therefore, fasting was recommended and practiced in conventional. Endocrinologists have reported their discovery that is treating epilepsy through starvation to the American Medical Association resolution. Even though fasting seemed a better medication for epilepsy, the seizures always returned after the fasting.

Dieting: Rollin Turner revised the study on diets and diabetes in 1921. He came to the conclusion that the liver produced three water molecules when they practiced fasting or when they consumed foods not rich in carbohydrates. Physicians, therefore, termed the 'Keto Diet' as nutrition that gave out increased levels of ketone molecules in the lifeblood after a high accumulation of calories and low levels of carbohydrates. Other physicians later formed 'the classic diet,' which involved rations of 1 gram of proteins for every kilogram of heaviness in children, ten to fifteen grams of carbohydrates daily, and the remaining fats from carbohydrates. There were positive effects associated with this type of dieting, that is, increased alertness, habits, and sleep. Unfavorable effects witnessed included vomiting caused by the significant amounts of ketone bodies. This type of dieting appeared favorable to the children as it improved seizure management on a diet. Though adults responded positively to the dieting as well, it was not as much as it did to the children.

The decline of anticonvulsants: Throughout the 1920 and 1930s, the keto diet was practiced, and that is the time where sedatives were the only anticonvulsant medicines available. However, this transformed when some doctors discovered new drugs, and every focus shifted on making more discoveries of new pills. By 1970, there were various drugs available to the doctors for the treatment of epileptic seizures, and this saw a decline in the usage of the keto diet as a medicine. Studies about the efficacy of the Keto diet declined until 1999, whereby the food was used to treat exceptional cases.

The MCT diet: Medium-chain triglycerides produced high levels of ketone molecules for every unit as compared to ordinary dietary calories. These triglycerides are easily absorbed and conveyed in the direction of the liver through the hepatic entryway system rather than the lymphatic coordination. The unembellished starch limitations made it hard for the parents to prepare appetizing diets which their kids would take, where approximately sixty percent of the fats came from the Medium-Chain Triglycerides. The MCT oil was then combined with skimmed milk and incorporated into the food: children with intractable seizures' health were improved through these diets.

The revival of the Keto diet: The Keto diet gained popularity in the United States of America in 1994 after Charlie Abraham's case was reported on NBC television. This young boy had uncontrollable epilepsy and did not get cured by any therapy that the doctors thought was the best. After practicing the keto diet, Charlie's average growth resumed. After Charlie's case was successfully treated, there were foundations aimed at studying more about this diet, and scientists began shifting their interests and focus on knowing more about the keto diet. By 2007, the keto diet had gained popularity in almost forty-five countries. Scientists and physicians concentrated on unleashing other possible uses of the keto diet rather than just treating epilepsy.

Keto diet's main aim is gaining more calories from proteins and oil rather than from carbohydrates. Your body's sugars get depleted, and this initiates fat breakdown, which leads to weight loss.

Advantages of the Keto Diet

Helps in losing weight: Keto diet helps in burning fats into energy, and this fat breakdown leads to weight loss. The diet encourages high intake of proteins, and this ensures that you are not hungry most of the time during the fasting period. Out of the many ways of losing weight and fasting, the keto diet recorded the best results.

Helps reduce acne: Acne is caused by several factors, including the type of diet you take and the amount of sugar in your menus. Keto diet encourages eating foods that have fewer carbohydrates, and this helps reduce sugar levels, which helps maintain a healthy body and skin.

Reduces cancer risks

Recent studies conclude that keto diets can be used in the prevention of any chances of cancer. It may be used as an alternative treatment for radiation in people who have the disease. Just like intermittent fasting, keto diet causes increased oxidative stress in cells containing cancer as it does to the healthy cells. Keto diet reduces sugar levels in your blood, a factor that helps in lowering insulin levels, a hormone commonly associated with cancer.

www.ingramcontent.com/pod-product-compliance
Lightning Source LLC
Chambersburg PA
CBHW071413210526
45465CB00001B/365

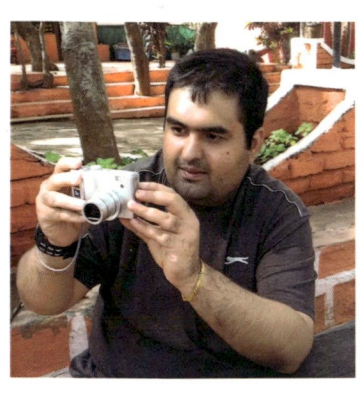
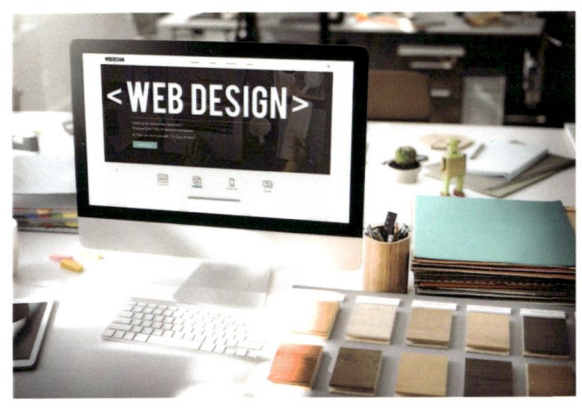

How to Start an Online Business from $32 a Month

Start a Web Design Business Blueprint Sell Your Blog and Websites Online

Smit Chacha

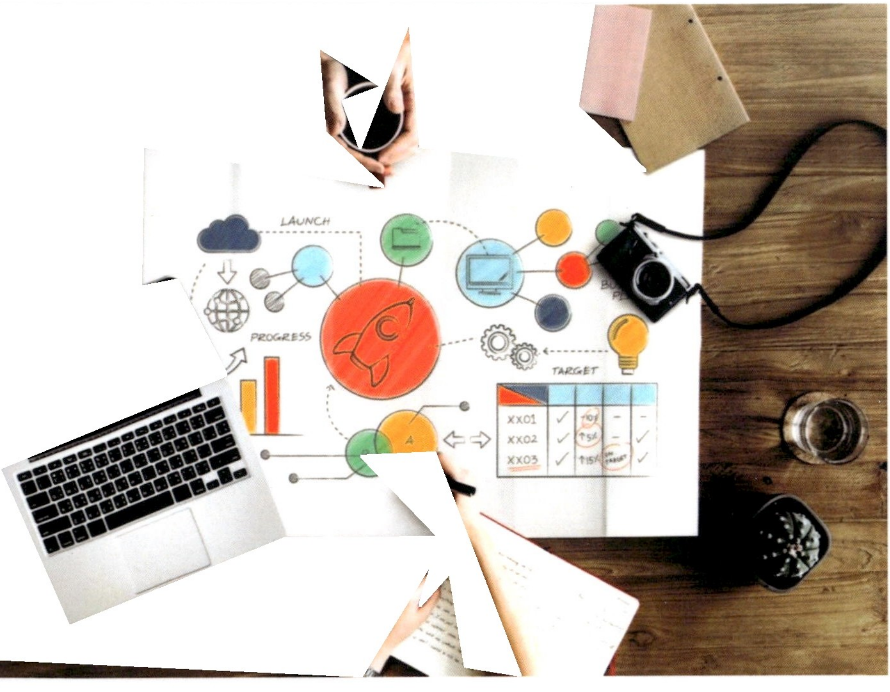